Readings in Speech Disfluency

Edited by
Gerald R. Moses, Ph.D.

MSS Information Corporation
655 Madison Avenue, New York, N.Y. 10021

CONTENTS

INTRODUCTION

The basic question of the relationship between stuttering
and normal disfluency has been approached by many authors. Others
have undertaken to establish normative data for each kind of
speech.

The purpose of this writing was to review some of the research pertaining to estimations of the frequency and severity
of stuttering, to present some of the important research pertaining to disfluency phenomena, and to suggest some clinical utility
from knowledge of these phenomena.

The reader, regardless of his theorectical position, may
find the following readings most helpful for understanding the
nature of disfluency. It is hoped that this understanding will
clarify the clinical picture of stuttering and lead to an appreciation of and toleration for normal disfluency.

Estimating the Frequency and
Severity of Stuttering

Johnson undertook to measure disfluency in stutterers and
nonstutterers.[5] His report contains the results of five researches.
One of the purposes of his research was to obtain normative and
comparative data with respect to rate and disfluency in the speech
and oral reading of adult male and female stutterers and non-
stutterers. His procedures refined earlier ones reported by
Bloodstein, et. al.,[1] Boehmler,[2] Darley,[3] and Tuthill.[11] These investigators tabulated individual moments of stuttering in various
ways and described the tonic and clonic nature of stuttering
blocks. Johnson went further to classify disfluency into eight
categories. He obtained normative data concerning speaking rate
and disfluency through analyzing tape-recorded samples of speaking and oral reading. His speakers were 100 male and 100 female
adult speakers, half of whom were stutterers and half of whom
were normal speakers.

Although to his ear adult stutterers showed to be more disfluent than adult nonstutterers, there was overlap among the distributions and frequencies of individual categories of disfluency.
The stutterers and the nonstutterers were indistinguishable with
respect to their scores for broken words and prolongations of
sounds. With respect to the repetition of words, approximately
20 per cent of the stutterers were more fluent than 30 to 40 per
cent of the nonstutterers. He presented normative data for each
category of disfluency for both groups of speakers. His work
ORIGINAL MANUSCRIPT.

7

served to precipitate many studies related to the measurement of disfluency.

Sander utilized Johnson's methodology for obtaining speech samples and employed another procedure for tallying "disfluent words."[8] He considered a word to be disfluent if it involved prolonged sounds, was classified as a broken word, was involved in a sound, syllable, or word repetition, or was interrupted by an interjection. Words preceded by interjections or involved in repetitions of phrases were not counted as disfluent words.

An investigation of disfluency in the speech of adult male stutterers as related to ratings of severity of stuttering was conducted by Young.[13] He reported that ratings by listeners of the severity of stuttering were related to the rate of utterance and to the number of words in relation to which a part-word repetition, a sound prolongation, a broken utterance, or unusual stress was observed, a word being counted only once no matter how often these types of behavior were observed during its production. Young called the disfluencies which he defined in this way "repetitions." These repetitions are the same as the disfluent words of Sander. Boehmler found that repetitions of sounds or syllables were classified by observers as stuttering more often than were other kinds of disfluency, while revisions and interjections were judged to be stuttering less often than were other disfluencies. Williams and Kent reported that their observers usually classified repetitions of syllables and prolongations of sounds as instances of stuttering, revisions as nonstuttered speech.[12]

8

In another study concerning listener reaction to disfluency, Giolas and Williams found that kindergarten children and ones' of the second grade were more accepting of interjections of vowel sounds than of syllable repetitions.[4]   Three principal procedures seem to be recommended by the foregoing researches for analyzing speech samples of stutterers. First, all disfluencies may be tabulated and classified in the categories described by Johnson. Second, analysis of samples of speech may be made in terms of Sanders' disfluent words. Third, a single category of disfluency, made up of what Young called repetitions, may be used to assess the frequency of stuttering. Normative and comparative data pertaining to these three kinds of analysis and the results based on the foregoing researches are reported by Johnson, Darley, and Spriestersbach.[6]

One approach to the assessment of the severity of stuttering led to a rating scale. Lewis and Sherman measured the apparent severity of stuttering in terms of the estimated degree of difficulty at the moment of stuttering rather than in terms of stuttering per unit of time.[7]   They presented 240 phonographically recorded speech samples to two groups of students of elementary psychology and to a panel of experienced judges of disfluent speech. The samples were rated by all of the listeners on a nine-point equal-appearing-intervals scale. Thirty-three nine-second samples representing the full range of severity from very mild to very severe were selected for use in training clinicians to recognize the levels of severity of stuttering. The scale became known as The Iowa Scale of Severity of Stuttering.

Sherman assessed the reliability of the Iowa Scale of
Severity of Stuttering by utilizing the nine-point equal-appearing-
intervals scale of severity to train 11 observers.[9] These observers then assigned scale values for levels of severity for 12
five-minute samples of stuttered speech. She concluded that con-
secutive judgments at short intervals by trained observers is
experimentally and clinically useful for assigning rank-order
positions of severity to samples of continuous stuttered speech.
In another study, Sherman determined that individual observers
were reliable in rating the severity of stuttering.[10] She also
found that scale values of severity of stuttering derived from
ratings by individual observers at 10-second intervals on three-
minute speech samples were fairly precise with respect to placing
the samples in relative positions along the severity dimension.
She further concluded that intensive training had no important
effect upon the reliability of severity ratings.

Young and Prather found that ratings of the severity of stuttering during 20 seconds of speech were comparable to ratings of
the total samples from which the segments were selected.[14] Young,
in another study, obtained ratings of severity of tape-recorded
samples of the speech of 50 adult stutterers. He played back the
recordings for three groups of listeners who were stutterers,
speech clinicians, and laymen. The listeners rated the samples
of speech on a nine-point equal-appearing-intervals scale. Twenty-
four hundred ratings of severity of stuttering were obtained from
the 48 listeners. A comparison of these ratings for the three

groups of listeners showed that the stutterers rated themselves
as more severe than did speech clinicians and laymen; also that
speech clinicians rated the stutterers as more severe than did
the laymen.

An advantage of rating scales is that they provide a degree
of uniformity and comparability among judgments. A scale of severity can provide for distinguishing mild from severe stuttering, or
mild from moderate or severe stuttering, and even finer distinctions.

Johnson, Darley, and Spriestersbach modified the Iowa Scale
of Severity of Stuttering. They introduced a seven-point scale.
This retains the values of an equal-appearing-intervals scale and
allows relatively greater specific description of each of the scale
values than does the nine-point one. The description of each scale
value pertains to the frequency of stuttered words relative to all
of the words spoken, the amount of detectable tension in the speech
sample, the duration of individual moments of stuttering, and the
amount of apparent distracting sounds or movements.

Gerald R. Moses

REFERENCES

1. Bloodstein, Oliver, William Jaeger, and Jack Tureen. "A
    Study of the Diagnosis of Stuttering by Parents of Stut-
    terers and Nonstutterers." Journal of Speech and Hearing
    Disorders, XVII (1952), 308-315.

2. Boehmler, Richard. "Listener Responses to Nonfluencies."
    Journal of Speech and Hearing Research, I (1958), 132-141.

3. Darley, Frederic L. "A Normative Study of Oral Reading
    Rate." Unpublished M.A. thesis, University of Iowa, 1939.

4. Giolas, Thomas G. and Dean E. Williams. "Childrens' Reac-
    tions to Nonfluencies in Adult Speech." Journal of Speech
    and Hearing Research, I (1958), 86-93.

5. Johnson, Wendell. "Measurements of Oral Reading and Speak-
    ing Rate and Disfluency of College-Age Male and Female
    Stutterers and Nonstutterers." Journal of Speech and Hear-
    ing Disorders, Monograph Supplement VIII (1961), 1-20.

6. Johnson, Wendell, Frederic L. Darley, and Duane C. Spriesters-
    bach. Diagnostic Methods in Speech Pathology. New York:
    Harper and Row Publishers, 1963.

7. Lewis, Don and Dorothy Sherman. "Measuring the Severity of
    Stuttering." Journal of Speech and Hearing Disorders, XVI
    (1951), 320-326.

8. Sander, Eric K. "Reliability of the Iowa Speech Disfluency
    Test." Journal of Speech and Hearing Disorders, Monograph
    Supplement VIII (1961), 21-30.

9. Sherman, Dorothy. "Clinical and Experimental Use of the
    Iowa Scale of Severity of Stuttering." Journal of Speech
    and Hearing Disorders, XVII (1952), 316-320.

10. Sherman, Dorothy. "Reliability and Utility of Individual
    Ratings of Severity and Audible Characteristics of Stutter-
    ing." Journal of Speech and Hearing Disorders, XX (1955),
    11-16.

11. Tuthill, Curtis, "A Quantitative Study of Extensional Meaning
    with Special Reference to Stuttering." Speech Monographs,
    XIII (1946), 81-98.

12. Williams, Dean E. and Louise R. Kent. "Listener Evaluations
    of Speech Interruptions." Journal of Speech and Hearing
    Research, I (1958), 124-131.

13. Young, Martin A. "Predicting Ratings of Severity of Stuttering." <u>Journal</u> <u>of</u> <u>Speech</u> <u>and</u> <u>Hearing</u> <u>Disorders</u>, Monograph Supplement VII (1961), 31-54.

14. Young, Martion A. and Elizabeth Moodie Prather. "Measuring Severity of Stuttering Using Short Segments of Speech." <u>Journal</u> <u>of</u> <u>Speech</u> <u>and</u> <u>Hearing</u> <u>Research</u>, V (1962), 256-262.

A Study Of The Diagnosis Of Stuttering By Parents Of Stutterers And Non-Stutterers

Oliver Bloodstein

William Jaeger

Jack Tureen

THIS STUDY was chiefly concerned with the question of whether parents of stutterers, if given the opportunity to express judgments about the recorded speech of a number of young children, would make diagnoses of stuttering more frequently than a group of parents of non-stutterers. It was designed to afford a partial test of Johnson's 'diagnosogenic' theory of stuttering (4, 5, 6, 7).

According to this theory, stuttering has its onset, for the most part, when children are taught by over-anxious adults to feel tense and fearful about their normal nonfluencies and consequently begin to struggle and strain in an effort to avoid them. To summarize Johnson's own concise statement of his theory, practically all stutterers are first diagnosed as such by a layman, usually a parent; what these laymen diagnose as stuttering is usually the normal nonfluency

of early childhood; stuttering as a disorder develops not before but after diagnosis, and the diagnosis, together with the unfavorable evaluations and pressures which it tends to involve, is one of its most important causes (5, 6). Parents are particularly likely to diagnose the normal speech hesitancies of their children as stuttering if they have unrealistically high and rigid standards of child behavior in general, or if a background of stuttering in the family has led them to anticipate and fear stuttering in their children (6):

> . . . these statements are not meant to imply that all children speak with equal fluency, nor that various biological and environmental influences are not more or less conducive to nonfluency (note the use of this term instead of 'stuttering') in 'normally speaking' children. . . (4)

The issue raised by Johnson is whether any children, before they have acquired feelings of self-consciousness or anxiety about the way they speak, exhibit nonfluency which is to be sharply differentiated from the speech hesitancies of most normal youngsters—in short, whether such a speech disorder as 'primary stuttering' (1) exists.

Johnson's theory of stuttering will be recognized to involve essentially three assumptions:

Oliver Bloodstein (Ph.D., Iowa, 1948) is Instructor in Speech, Brooklyn College, William Jaeger (M.A., Brooklyn, 1952) is Speech Therapist, Goldwater Memorial Hospital, and Jack Tureen (M.A., Brooklyn, 1952) is Instructor in Speech, Long Island University. Paul B. Williams, Assistant Professor of Speech, Brooklyn College, cooperated in the study by making available the recording facilities of the Brooklyn College Radio Laboratory.

JOURNAL OF SPEECH AND HEARING DISORDERS, 1952, Vol. pp. 308-315.

1. Most normal young children speak with a considerable amount of repetition and other breaks in fluency.

2. Adults differ in their standards of fluency, and some react to the hesitant speech of children with unusual intolerance.

3. Children who are penalized for normal nonfluencies are likely to develop stuttering.

The first of these assumptions has been tested and substantially confirmed by Davis (2).[1] The second was the special concern of this study. Some previous work relevant to this assumption was done by Tuthill (9), who asked groups of speech clinicians, stutterers, and laymen to designate all stuttered words observed in phonograph and sound film recordings of the speech of several adult stutterers and non-stutterers. Tuthill found that these subjects had disagreed markedly as to the specific speech manifestations which were regarded as stuttering and as to the number of stutterings which had occurred.

The study reported here dealt with differences in adult standards of fluency in somewhat more direct relation to the assumption at issue. By determining how strongly parents of young stutterers were disposed to make the diagnosis of stuttering it was the aim of this study to demonstrate to what extent they revealed the specific behavior which Johnson believes to be crucially involved in the onset of stuttering.

Procedure

The subjects were 48 parents, consisting of 24 married couples. Half of

these were parents of children who had been referred to the Brooklyn College Community Speech and Hearing Center as stutterers. These children ranged in age from 3.5 to eight, and had a median age of six. The remaining parents had children, ranging in age from four to ten, who had never been regarded as stutterers. The two groups of parents were approximately similar in age, both groups ranging from 25 to 43.

In addition, 12 subjects were used in making recordings of the spontaneous speech of children. Of these, six were non-stutterers and six were regarded by their parents as stutterers.[2] This group consisted of 10 boys and two girls, ranging from age 3.5 to age eight, with a median age of 5.5. A series of picture cards was presented to each child, and a tape recording was made as he responded to instructions to 'tell a story' about each. The tape was then edited to provide 12 two-minute samples of continuous speech, one from each child.[3]

This recording was played to small groups of parents on several successive occasions until all 48 subjects had been tested. At each session numbered sheets of paper were distributed, and the subjects received standard instructions to indicate, after listening to each recorded speech sample, whether the child just heard was a stutterer or

[1] Davis found that the average child in a group of 62 two- to six-year-olds exhibited 45 instances of syllable, word or phrase repetition per thousand words of spontaneous speech. This would probably amount to several repetitions per minute of running speech, assuming the slowest reasonable speaking rates.

[2] Any attempt to justify the description of these six children as stutterers is unnecessary in view of the fact that parents, not children, were the objects of study. For convenience, the recordings of the speech of these six children will be referred to as stutterers' recordings. The same considerations are involved in referring to the subjects in the experimental group as parents of stutterers.

[3] The parents of five of the stutterers and three of the non-stutterers whose speech was recorded served as subjects in the study.

TABLE 1. Diagnoses of stuttering made by parents of stutterers and non-stutterers in response to two-minute recorded samples of the spontaneous speech of six stuttering and six non-stuttering children.

	Parents of Stutterers	Parents of Non-Stutterers
Both Parents (24 each group)		
Mean	5.1	2.9
Median	6.0	2.5
Range	0-9	0-7
S. D.	2.76	1.80
Mothers (12 each group)		
Mean	5.2	2.7
Median	6.5	2.5
Range	0-9	0-6
S. D.	3.02	1.69
Fathers (12 each group)		
Mean	5.1	3.1
Median	6.0	2.5
Range	0-8	1-7
S. D.	2.47	1.89

a normal speaker. Precautions were taken to insure independent responses. No other instructions were given.

Results

The essential findings are summarized in Table 1. Parents of stutterers will be seen to have made a median score of 6.0 diagnoses of stuttering as compared to a median score of 2.5 for their controls. This difference is significant at the 0.1 per cent level of confidence, t being 4.08. The corresponding difference in means is somewhat smaller as a result of the fact that a few parents in each group had scores markedly contrary to the group trends. Table 1 also contains data relating to the mothers and to the fathers of stutterers and non-stutterers. Tests of significance of the differences among the various means are summarized in Table 2.

Table 2 shows that the only non-significant differences were those obtained in comparing mothers with fathers. Not only did mothers and fathers score approximately alike as groups, but, to some extent, so did married couples. This tendency was especially conspicuous among parents of non-stutterers, whose scores showed a statistically significant product-moment correlation of .76. The correlation between parents of stutterers was not significantly greater than zero, r being .34, but the exclusion of two extreme cases of disparity between a husband and wife results in a significant r of .72.[4] These relationships are shown graphically in Figure 1.

Figure 1 permits a ready comparison of the joint scores of parental pairs in the experimental group with those of the control group. If scores of four or less are arbitrarily considered 'tolerant' and all higher scores 'intolerant,' it will be seen that in seven cases in which both the mother and the father scored intolerantly all

[4]Values of significant correlation coefficients for small samples are given by Lindquist (8).

16

TABLE 2. Summary of tests of significance of the differences between groups and between sub-groups of parents in mean number of diagnoses of stuttering.

	t	Significance Level
Parents of Stutterers and Parents of Non-Stutterers	3.25	1%
Mothers of Stutterers and Mothers of Non-Stutterers	2.37	5%
Fathers of Stutterers and Fathers of Non-Stutterers	2.13	5%
Mothers of Stutterers and Fathers of Stutterers	0.09	Not at 90%
Mothers of Non-Stutterers and Fathers of Non-Stutterers	0.98	40%

but one of the children stutter. In 12 cases in which both parents were tolerant all but three of the children speak normally. In the remaining five cases in which either a mother or a father is intolerant there are three stuttering children. Figure 1 may also be interpreted from the point of view of the stuttering and non-stuttering children of these parents. Of the 12 stutterers six have intolerant mothers and fathers, two have intolerant fathers, one has an intolerant mother, and the remaining three have tolerant mothers and fathers. Of the 12 non-stutterers nine have tolerant mothers and fathers, one has a moderately intolerant mother, one has a moderately intolerant father, and one has two intolerant parents.

All of the foregoing results have dealt with subjects' responses to the 12 recordings considered as a whole. It will be recalled that half of these samples were furnished by supposedly stuttering children, and half by children who were regarded by their parents as normal speakers. The data were analyzed to provide separate scores for each parent representing the number of non-stutterers' recordings and the number of stutterers' recordings to which he had reacted with

a diagnosis of stuttering. It was found that in listening to the six samples of normal speech the average parent of a stutterer made 1.8 diagnoses of stuttering, as compared to 0.9 made by

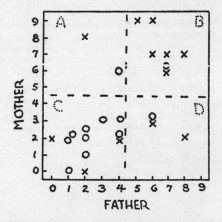

FIGURE 1. Scatter diagram of joint scores of 12 pairs of parents of stutterers and 12 pairs of parents of non-stutterers. The scores represent the number of diagnoses of stuttering made in response to recorded samples of the spontaneous speech of 12 young children. The quadrants are based on an arbitrary division of the scale into 'tolerant' and 'intolerant' scores: A, intolerant mother and tolerant father; B, intolerant mother and father; C, tolerant mother and father; D, tolerant mother and intolerant father; X, parents of a stutterer; O, parents of a non-stutterer.

17

the average parent of a non-stutterer. This difference is significant at the 2 per cent level of confidence, t being 2.44. In response to the six recordings of stuttering children the mean scores were 3.3 for parents of stutterers and 2.0 for parents of non-stutterers, a difference significant at the 1 per cent level, t being 3.03. It may be concluded that the parents of stutterers exceeded their controls in diagnosing the non-stuttering, as well as the stuttering children as stutterers.

A more detailed comparison of the two groups of parents may be made by examining their responses to each of the 12 recordings considered individually. Such a comparison is made in Table 3. While the proportions shown are based on groups of subjects too small to permit statistical analysis, a tendency is evident almost throughout the series for parents of stutterers to make a larger number of diagnoses of stuttering than parents of non-stutterers.

It has been mentioned that several of the children used in making the speech recordings had parents who served as subjects. As a consequence, 10 of the 24 parents of stutterers and six of the 24 parents of non-stutterers heard, and may have identified their own children in listening to the recordings. It is of interest that when the scores of these subjects are eliminated the findings do not differ essentially from those which have been reported for the 48 subjects as a whole. The 14 parents of stutterers who did not hear their own children had a mean score of 5.9 diagnoses of stuttering in response to the 12 recorded speech samples. The 18 parents of non-stutterers who did not hear their own children had a mean score of 3.0. The difference is significant at the 0.1 per cent level of confidence, t being 3.71.

Discussion

The results of this study accord so well with a 'diagnosogenic' theory of stuttering that it is hardly possible to discuss them adequately without essentially restating much of what Johnson has already written (4, 5, 6, 7). Of basic interest is the finding that the parents of stutterers made a larger number of diagnoses of stuttering than a group of parents of non-stutterers. It is particularly relevant to the questions raised in this study that they applied this description to the speech of the non-stuttering children significantly more often than did their controls. The inference can be drawn that an unusual number of these parents have rather high expectations regarding the fluency of young children, and are consequently inclined

TABLE 3. Number of diagnoses of stuttering made by parents of stutterers and non-stutterers in response to recordings of spontaneous speech of 12 children. (N, each group=24)

| | Recordings (in order presented) | | | | | | | | | | | |
	1	2	3*	4*	5	6*	7	8*	9	10	11*	12*
Parents of Stutterers	13	9	17	10	6	4	1	14	7	7	14	20
Parents of Non-Stutterers	5	3	14.5†	5	5	0	0	15	6	3	2	11

*Stutterer.

†One parent of a non-stutterer was unable to form a judgment about recording 3. Her response was counted as one-half.

to react to them as stutterers more readily than is the average parent in the control group.

The implications of this statement must be developed with some care. The possibility will be recognized that the perfectionism of these parents resulted from, rather than caused their children's stuttering. It must be kept in mind for this reason that this study does not demonstrate the effect of high standards of fluency on the speech of children. It demonstrates only that such high standards exist. This is, however, of more than academic interest. That the mother of a stutterer is distressed, anxious, and generally concerned about her child's speech is to be expected. But to find that she may also be more inclined to diagnose the normal speech hesitations of another child as stuttering, whether for this reason or for any other, is a very different matter and is of much greater significance. If an individual may acquire unrealistic standards of fluency as a reaction to his child's stuttering it is not far to the inference that he may acquire them also as a reaction to the stuttering of his father, his brother, or any other member of his family, or as a reaction to his own stuttering. Furthermore, if a family background of stuttering may foster these attitudes there is no logical bar to the inference that they may arise from other sources of perfectionism. The point is that people apparently do acquire such attitudes. The single fact of basic importance which this study demonstrated is that, whatever the reasons involved, an individual may regard as exceptional and defective the very same childhood speech patterns which others evidently consider quite normal.

What the consequences of such an evaluation may be is largely a matter of the role which penalty, fear, and avoidance play in the development of stuttering. The work of Froeschels (3), Bluemel (1), Van Riper (10), and others has lent strong support to the belief that the chronic tensions characteristic of developed stuttering result from penalty in various forms. What has been widely assumed, however, is that such penalty is practically always 'justified,' in a sense, by the presence of an abnormal degree of nonfluency. Bluemel termed this 'primary stuttering.' While various constitutional and emotional theories have been offered to account for the onset of primary stuttering, it is believed to develop into a serious disorder, generally speaking, only if the child is made to feel guilty and apprehensive about the interruptions in his speech (10, 11). On the face of it, there seems little reason to suppose that the consequences of penalty for normal nonfluencies would differ markedly from the consequences of penalty for 'primary stuttering.' It need hardly be said that the child is incapable of making such a distinction.

The chief question raised by the results of this study is whether such a distinction can be made at all. The assumption involved in the concept of primary stuttering is that any nonfluency so excessive and conspicuous that it is regarded with concern by a parent deserves to be regarded as an abnormality by the speech pathologist. This would imply that parents agree fairly well on what they find to be 'excessive' and 'conspicuous.' In this study two groups of parents revealed a remarkable difference of opinion as to the meaning of such a description. The crucial implication of this finding is that the extent to which a child's nonfluency is excessive or conspicuous is determined not solely by the amount of repetition in his speech but also, to a significant degree, by who is listening. In so far as this is true, the term 'primary stuttering' loses much of its meaning.

This is not to say that some children are not, on the whole, less fluent than others, or that this is of no consequence so far as the onset of stuttering is concerned. It should be recalled that three married couples showing rather tolerant reactions to the recordings have children who stutter, while one couple who made a large number of diagnoses of stuttering has a child who speaks normally. In these instances one might be justified in attaching considerable importance to differences in the fluency of the children rather than to differences in the speech standards of the parents. A significant question would appear to be the relative influence which each of these factors has in determining the likelihood that children will come to be regarded as excessively nonfluent by their parents and made to feel tense and uncomfortable about interruptions in their speech. To the extent that this is a matter of how much they repeat and hesitate there would seem to be adequate reason for asking various other questions regarding the neurological, biochemical, psychosexual or other origins of these repetitions, or concerned with the interplay of predisposing and precipitating factors in their etiology. To the extent that parents' evaluations are at fault such questions are beside the point.

Exactly how large a part is played in the onset of stuttering by the evaluative factor is not revealed by the results of this study. That is plays some part is clearly suggested. If the findings do not allow the inference that extreme degrees of nonfluency may be safely ignored, neither do they permit the naive assumption that a child is distinctive in some way merely because his parents say he is a stutterer. While relevant questions may be asked concerning the conditions under which nonfluency varies, the concept of primary stuttering with its elaborate implications of abnormality would seem to be open to serious criticism.

Summary

As a partial test of Johnson's 'diagnosogenic' theory of stuttering, 24 parents of young stutterers and 24 parents of young non-stutterers were asked to diagnose as 'stuttering' or 'normal' the recorded spontaneous speech of six stuttering and six non-stuttering children. The following were the essential findings:

1. Parents of stutterers significantly exceeded parents of non-stutterers in the extent to which they diagnosed both the stuttering and non-stuttering children as stutterers.

2. Among parents of stutterers as well as among parents of non-stutterers, mothers and fathers as groups did not differ significantly in the number of diagnoses of stuttering which they made.

3. There was a tendency for married couples to score somewhat alike, especially among parents of non-stutterers.

The results are consistent with a 'diagnosogenic' theory of stuttering. In view of the findings, the usefulness of the term 'primary stuttering' appears open to some doubt. Assuming that penalty for speech interruptions is instrumental in the development of stuttering, parental standards of fluency would seem to play a definite part in its onset.

References

1. BLUEMEL, C. S. Primary and secondary stammering. *Quart. J. Speech*, 18, 1932, 187-200.

2. DAVIS, D. M. The relation of repetitions in the speech of young children to certain measures of language maturity and situational factors: Part I. *JSD*, 4, 1939, 303-318.
3. FROESCHELS, E. Beitrage·zur Symptomatologie des Stotterns. *Mschr. Ohrenheilk.*, 55, 1921, 1109-1112.
4. HAHN, E. F. *Stuttering: Significant Theories and Therapies.* Stanford Univ., Calif.: Stanford Univ. Press. 1943.
5. JOHNSON, W. *People in Quandaries: The Semantics of Personal Adjustment.* New York: Harper, 1946.
6. JOHNSON, W., BROWN, S. F., CURTIS, J. F., EDNEY, C. W. AND KEASTER, J. *Speech Handicapped School Children.* New York: Harper, 1946.
7. JOHNSON, W. et al. A study of the onset and development of stuttering. *JSD*, 7, 1942, 251-257.
8. LINDQUIST, E. F. *Statistical Analysis in Educational Research.* Boston: Houghton Mifflin, 1940.
9. TUTHILL, C. A quantitative study of extensional meaning with special reference to stuttering. *Speech Monogr.*, 13, 1946, 81-98.
10. VAN RIPER, C. *Speech Correction: Principles and Methods.* (Rev. ed.) New York: Prentice-Hall, 1947.
11. WEST, R., KENNEDY, L., CARR, A. AND BACKUS, O. *The Rehabilitation of Speech.* (Rev. ed.) New York: Harper, 1947.

Listener Responses To Non-Fluencies

Richard M. Boehmler

This experiment was concerned with studying speech responses which are extensionally designated as stuttering behavior. The main purposes were to investigate (1) the relationship between the rated severity of moments of non-fluency and the behavior of judges in labeling these speech phenomena as stuttering and (2) the relationship between the training of the judges and their behavior in the labeling process. Another purpose was to evaluate relationships between types of non-fluency and the behavior of judges in the labeling process.

Procedure

Selection of Speech Samples. Samples of non-fluencies were selected from short tape recordings of the speech of 90 college students, 60 non-stutterers and 30 stutterers. Each speech sample was approximately five seconds in length and contained only one moment of non-fluency. The selection was made to obtain a wide range of severity and different types of non-fluencies. The total selection consisted of 804 samples, 402 from

the speech of stutterers and 402 from the speech of non-stutterers.

The 804 samples were presented in random order to a group of 32 elementary psychology students. They rated the severity of each non-fluency on a seven-point equal-appearing intervals scale extending from *one*, for least severe, to *seven*, for most severe. A median scale value was obtained for each sample by the method described by Thurstone and Chave (6). Each of the two groups of samples was then divided into three sub-groups according to the obtained severity ratings. Samples with large Q-values or with median scale values near the points of division between two sub-groups were eliminated. The final selection consisted of six sub-groups of 100 samples each. The means of the obtained median scale values of the six sub-groups were as follows: 1.90 for mild samples from the speech of non-stutterers; 2.95 for average samples from the speech of non-stutterers; 4.13 for severe samples from the speech of non-stutterers; 2.45 for mild samples from the speech of stutterers; 4.20 for average samples from the speech of stutterers; 6.08 for severe samples from the speech of stutterers.

Judging of the Speech Samples. Three groups of judges which differed from each other in degree and in kind of training in stuttering

Richard M. Boehmler (Ph.D., State University of Iowa, 1953) is Assistant Professor of Speech Pathology and Audiology, Humboldt State College. This article is based on a doctoral dissertation completed under the direction of Professors Wendell Johnson and Dorothy Sherman.

JOURNAL OF SPEECH AND HEARING RESEARCH, 1958, Vol. 1, pp. 132-141.

TABLE 1. Summary of analysis of variance for evaluation of the frequency of stuttering label data.

Source of Variation	df	ss	ms	F *	p†
Between Subjects	29	25227.36			
Judges (J)	2	9801.35	4900.68	8.52	.005
error (b)	27	15536.01	575.41		
Within Subjects	150	157092.17			
Severity (S)	2	57033.75	28516.87	546.51	.001
Origin (O)	1	76590.94	76590.94	975.93	.001
SO	2	12530.52	6265.26	112.76	.001
SJ	4	798.18	199.54	15.29	.001
OJ	2	384.20	192.10	2.45	NS††
SOJ	4	11618.84	2904.72	52.28	.001
error (w)	135	7937.12	58.79		
error$_1$ (w)	54	2817.80	52.18		
error$_2$ (w)	27	2119.03	78.48		
error$_3$ (w)	54	3000.29	55.56		
Total	179	182429.53			

*F-ratios: $ms_J/ms_{error(b)}$; $ms_S/ms_{error_1(w)}$; $ms_O/ms_{error_2(w)}$; $ms_{SO}/ms_{error_3(w)}$; $ms_{SJ}/ms_{error_1(w)}$; $ms_{OJ}/ms_{error_2(w)}$; $ms_{SOJ}/ms_{error_3(w)}$
†p = point in the F-distribution
††Not significant

theory and therapy were selected. One group (Trained A) consisted of 10 graduate students in speech pathology who had had at least three semester hours of training in the area of stuttering and clinical experience with at least one stutterer at the State University of Iowa. Another group (Trained B) consisted of 10 staff members at the Institute of Logopedics who had had at least as much training and experience as the members of the Trained A group. The third group (Untrained) consisted of 10 elementary psychology students who had had no training in speech pathology.

The 600 samples were presented in random order by tape playback to each of the three groups of judges at three separate listening sessions. The judges were instructed to record S for each sample which seemed to contain an example of 'stuttering' and N for each sample which seemed to con-

TABLE 2. Mean frequencies of the stuttering label for six sub-groups of 100 non-fluencies each, judged by three groups of observers (1. Trained A, 2. Trained B and 3. Untrained).

Origin	Sub-groups	Judges			General Means	
		1	2	3	(Sub-groups)	(Origins)
Non-stutterers	Mild	12.8	27.0	10.9	16.9	
	Average	20.7	35.5	14.2	23.5	27.5
	Severe	43.8	54.5	28.2	42.2	
Stutterers	Mild	31.7	49.2	22.9	34.6	
	Average	76.5	83.9	65.4	75.3	68.6
	Severe	98.3	95.3	95.7	96.4	
(General Means)		47.3	57.6	39.6		

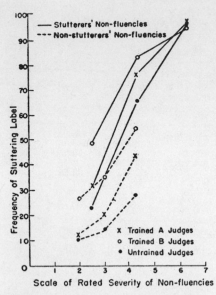

FIGURE 1. The trends of mean frequencies of the use of the stuttering label as a function of rated severity. Each plotted point represents the mean for 100 speech samples.

tain an example of 'non-stuttering' non-fluency.

Results

Frequency of Labeling. The measure for the frequency of labeling was the number of non-fluencies within any one sub-group of 100 speech samples labeled by one judge as 'stuttering.' The obtained data were evaluated by an analysis of variance described by Lindquist (5) and identified as Type VI. The analysis included three factors: (1) training of judges (Trained A, Trained B and Untrained); (2) origin of non-fluencies (from the speech of stutterers and from the speech of non-stutterers); and (3) severity of non-fluencies (mild, average and severe). A summary of the analysis is presented in

Table 1. Table 2 gives the mean frequency of labeling for each of the 18 combinations among classifications. The trend of frequency of labeling as a function of rated severity is represented graphically[1] for each of the three groups of judges for each origin in Figure 1.

Labeling in Relation to Groups of Judges. The judges differed from group to group in the mean frequency of application of the stuttering label. The trained B group did the most labeling, with a mean of 57.6 out of a possible 100. The Trained A group was next with a mean of 47.3. The Untrained group did the least amount of labeling with a mean of 39.6. The differences among these means were highly significant (See Table 1). These results provide evidence that individuals who differ in the degree and kind of training in speech pathology are likely to differ also in the frequency with which they apply the stuttering label. This confirms the finding by Tuthill (7) who reported that clinicians did more labeling than non-clinicians. Both the interaction of severity with training and the interaction of origin with training effects are significant. In other words, the differences among the groups of judges vary from one sub-group of non-fluencies to another and also from the speech of stutterers to the speech of non-stutterers. However, an examination of the data shows that the same rank order is retained for all groups of judges for the two origins and for all six sub-groups

---

[1]The graphical representation does not correspond exactly to the statistical analysis in that the abscissa represents scale values of rated severity. For purposes of statistical analysis the differences evaluated are between corresponding mild, average and severe categories.

of non-fluencies with the single exception of the severe samples from the speech of stutterers. In this instance the differences are very small. The change in rank order can thus be accounted for by the fact that the maximum possible frequency of labeling was being approached with high agreement among groups.

Labeling in Relation to Severity of Samples. The differences among the mean frequencies of labeling for the three severity sub-groups of non-fluency samples were highly significant for both origins (stuttering and non-stuttering) combined. The rank order indicated that the more severe the sample of non-fluency, the more likely it is to be labeled as stuttering. The rank order was from mild to average to severe for all groups of judges and for both origins of the samples. Apparently, severity of the non-fluency being judged is a major determinant for application of the stuttering label.

Labeling in Relation to Origin of Non-Fluencies. The stuttering label was applied more frequently to the samples taken from the speech of stutterers than to those taken from the speech of non-stutterers, as shown

in Figure 1. The differences between the two origins varied somewhat with the level of severity, but in all cases the samples in the sub-groups from the stutterers were labeled as stuttering more frequently than were the samples in the corresponding groups from the non-stutterers. This difference can be accounted for in part by the generally greater severity of the samples from the stutterers. However, Figure 1 also shows that the stuttering label was more frequently applied to samples from the speech of stutterers than to samples from the speech of non-stutterers even when the samples from the two origins were of approximately equal mean severity. For example, although comparable in rated severity, the average samples of non-fluency from the speech of stutterers were more frequently labeled as stuttering than were the severe samples of non-fluency from the speech of non-stutterers. Apparently factors other than the rated severity of the moment of non-fluency influence the labeling process.

Labeling in Relation to the Type of Non-Fluency. A fourth factor, type of non-fluency, was investigated by

TABLE 3. Frequency of each type of non-fluency within each sub-group of experimental speech samples.

Types of Non-fluencies	From the Speech of Non-stutterers			From the Speech of Stutterers		
	Mild	Average	Severe	Mild	Average	Severe
Interjections	6	7	11	5	8	9
Repetitions of Sounds or Syllables	32	17	6	19	24	25
Repetitions of Words	27	19	11	12	11	5
Repetitions of Phrases	9	10	5	12	3	0
Revisions	7	17	5	2	0	0
Prolongations	5	2	0	13	4	6
Mixtures	14	26	57	21	39	55
Others	0	3	5	16	11	0
Total	100	100	100	100	100	100

means of a chi-square test of independence. The categories, or types of non-fluencies, were as follows: (1) interjected sounds, instances of any extraneous sound such as 'uh' or 'er' which was distinct from sounds associated with the repetitions of an initial sound or syllable; (2) repetitions of sounds or syllables; (3) repetitions of single words; (4) repetitions of phrases, instances of any repetition of more than one word in which no revision was made in the course of the repetition; (5) revisions, instances in which the wording of a phrase was modified by changing at least one word with a resultant change in the meaning of the phrase; (6) prolongations, instances of any apparent prolongation of a sound at the beginning or end of a word, or within a word; (7) mixtures, instances of any complex moment of non-fluency which consisted of more than one type, such as a repetition of a sound within a repetition of a word; (8) others, instances of an explosive, a pause, a broken word, or an interrupted phrase (these occurred relatively infrequently and were grouped to avoid too small theoretical frequencies for a chi-square test). The

TABLE 4. Frequencies of non-fluency types in 400 samples of speech, 100 from each of four subgroups, average samples and severe samples from the speech of non-stutterers and mild samples and average samples from the speech of stutterers.

Type of Non-Fluency	Frequency Below Median*	Frequency Above Median*	Total
Word Repetitions	24 (26.5)†	29 (26.5)	53
Sound or Syllable Repetitions	21 (33)	45 (33)	66
Phrase Repetitions	19 (15)	11 (15)	30
Mixtures	68 (71.5)	75 (71.5)	143
Revisions	18 (12)	6 (12)	24
Interjections	20 (15.5)	11 (15.5)	31
Prolongations	13 (9.5)	6 (9.5)	19
All Others	17 (17)	17 (17)	34
Total	200	200	400

Chi-square ($df=7$) = 21.83, significant beyond one per cent level.

*The non-fluencies were dichotomized as Below Median and Above Median with reference to the number of judges applying the stuttering label.

†Values within parentheses are the theoretical or expected frequencies.

distribution of samples among categories is given in Table 3.

To study the relationship between frequency of labeling and the type of non-fluency, it was necessary to control the influence of severity by using only four sub-groups. When all six sub-groups were included, the average rated severities of samples from non-stutterers and stutterers were 2.99 and 4.23, respectively. For the combined average and severe samples from the speech of non-stutterers and for the combined mild and average samples from the speech of stutterers, the averaged rated severities were approximately the same, 3.54 and 3.31, respectively. The mild samples from the speech of non-stutterers and the severe samples from the speech of stutterers were thus omitted from this part of the analysis.

The measure was the number of judges who labeled a non-fluency as an example of stuttering. Since there were 30 judges, the measure could vary from zero to 30. The median of the measures for the 200 samples from the speech of stutterers was 16.5, and the median of the measures for the 200 samples from the speech of non-stutterers was 8.77. These median values were used as the reference points for dichotomizing the samples. If the number of judges labeling a sample as stuttering exceeded 16.5 for the samples from the speech of non-stutterers or 8.77 for the samples from the speech of stutterers, the sample was classified as reported in Table 4 as 'Above Median.' If the number of judges labeling a given sample fell below the appropriate reference value, it was classified as 'Below Median.'

To test the hypothesis that the number of judges labeling a given sample was independent of the type of non-fluency, a chi-square was computed from the data presented in Table 4. A highly significant result indicated that the number of judges labeling a given sample as stuttering was related to the type of non-fluency contained within the sample. In the category of repetition of sounds and syllables, 45 samples (17 of 23 from non-stutterers and 28 of 43 from stutterers) were above the medians and 21 were below. The evidence thus indicates that samples containing sound or syllable repetitions are likely to be labeled as stuttering. This may be one reason that the non-fluencies from the speech of stutterers were more frequently labeled as stuttering than were the non-fluencies from the speech of non-stutterers. More of the samples from stutterers contained sound or syllable repetition than did the samples from the non-stutterers.

The mixed samples were approximately equally distributed above and below the median frequency values of application of the stuttering label. However, 53 of the 143 mixed samples contained sound or syllable repetitions and 79 per cent of these 53 samples were above the medians. Also, among the mild samples from the speech of non-stutterers, which were not included in the chi-square test, five of the six samples most frequently labeled as stuttering contained sound or syllable repetitions. Thus, there is some further evidence beyond that provided by the significant chi-square value that samples containing sound or syllable repetitions are likely to be labeled as stuttering. Furthermore, severity could be ruled out as an important factor since the average severity, 3.43, of all samples in the four sub-groups was approximately the same as the average severity, 3.35, of the samples containing sound and syllable repetitions.

Revisions also may have contributed to the difference between samples from the speech of non-stutterers and those from the speech of stutterers with respect to the frequency of the stuttering label. As indicated in Table 4, there were three times more revision samples below than above the median. As indicated in Table 3, there were 22 revision samples from the speech of non-stutterers as compared with two from the speech of stutterers. Other categories may also have contributed to the difference between the two origins, but small frequencies preclude further interpretation with regard to the importance of various types of non-fluencies.

Table 4 shows that samples containing interjections were likely not to be labeled as stuttering. This tendency did not contribute importantly to the difference in the frequency of use of the stuttering label between the samples from the speech of non-stutterers and those from the speech of stutterers, since the samples were about equally distributed between the two origins (See Table 3).

On the basis of the results obtained, the assumption may be made that types of non-fluency have some effect on the labeling process. Also warranted is the assumption that non-fluencies consisting of syllable or sound repetition are labeled as stuttering more frequently than are non-fluencies of other types, and non-fluencies consisting of revisions or interjections are labeled less frequently.

Extensional Agreement Index. The criterion measures used to quantify extensional agreement were obtained by the following formula:

$$EAI = (2X-n)/n$$

where n represents the number of judges in a group and X is the number within a group who consider a particular sample of non-fluency to be an example of stuttering. This measure has been presented and discussed by Johnson (4).

Three measures of extensional agreement were available for each sample, one for each group of judges. The data were evaluated by the same method used for the frequency of labeling. The analysis included the same three factors: (1) training of judges (Trained A, Trained B and Untrained); (2) origin of non-fluencies

TABLE 5. Mean extensional agreement indexes for application of the stuttering label for six subgroups of 100 non-fluencies each, judged by three groups of observers (1. Trained A, 2. Trained B and 3. Untrained).

| Origin | Sub-groups | Judges | | | General Means | |
		1	2	3	(Sub-groups)	(Origins)
	Mild	76.8	56.6	76.6	70.0	
Non-stutterers	Average	63.6	45.2	72.2	60.0	60.0
	Severe	48.0	44.2	57.4	49.9	
	Mild	51.2	47.0	62.2	53.5	
Stutterers	Average	64.4	75.2	52.0	63.9	70.7
	Severe	97.8	94.0	92.4	94.7	
(General Means)		67.0	60.4	68.6		

TABLE 6. Summary of analysis of variance for evaluation of extensional agreement index data.

Source of Variation	df	ss	ms	F*	p†
Between Samples	599	1177697.78			
Severity (S)	2	43832.45	21916.22	22.4	.001
Origin (O)	1	51842.00	51842.00	52.9	.001
SO	2	326689.33	163344.66	166.8	.001
error (b)	594	581596.66	979.12		
Within Samples	1200	833866.89			
Judges (J)	2	22935.78	11467.87	19.3	.001
JS	4	14528.79	3632.19	6.1	.001
JO	2	40758.67	20379.33	34.2	.001
JOS	4	47960.33	11990.08	20.1	.001
error (w)	1188	707683.32	595.68		
Total	1799	1899413.12			

*F-ratios: $ms_S/ms_{error(b)}$; $ms_O/ms_{error(b)}$; $ms_{SO}/ms_{error(b)}$; $ms_J/ms_{error(w)}$; $ms_{JS}/ms_{error(w)}$; $ms_{JO}/ms_{error(w)}$; $ms_{JOS}/ms_{error(w)}$
†p = point in the F-distribution

(from the speech of stutterers and from the speech of non-stutterers); and (3) severity of non-fluencies (mild, average and severe). Table 5 presents the mean extensional agreement index for each of the 18 combinations among the factor classifica-

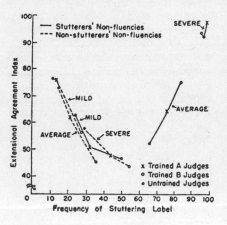

FIGURE 2. The trends of mean frequencies of the use of the stuttering label as a function of the extensional agreement index. Each plotted point represents the mean for 100 speech samples.

tions. A summary of the analysis is given in Table 6. All F-test results were highly significant. The relationships among the factors are apparently complex, and the significant interactions preclude any very meaningful interpretation of the results of the analysis. Examination of the means in Table 5, however, makes apparent that judges agreed best on the severe non-fluencies of stutterers and next best on the mild non-fluencies of non-stutterers. They agreed least on the severe non-fluencies of non-stutterers, with the next poorest agreement on the mild non-fluencies of stutterers.

Figure 2 shows the average extensional agreement index plotted against the corresponding frequency of application of the stuttering label for each of the 18 combinations of groups of speech samples with groups of judges. Examination of the figure makes readily apparent that the trends over groups of judges were highly similar for four groups of speech samples—the mild, average and severe non-stuttering samples and the mild

29

stuttering samples. In each instance the Untrained Judges applied the stuttering label least frequently and had the highest agreement while the Trained B Judges applied the label the most frequently and had the lowest agreement. The trend is the reverse for the average stuttering samples, the groups remaining in the same order with respect to frequency of application of the stuttering label but with higher agreement accompanying increase of frequency. For the severe stuttering samples, as might be expected, both the agreement and the frequency of labeling are quite high for all three groups of judges and any trend appears negligible.

Discussion

The positive relationship between the frequency of the label 'stuttering' and the severity of the moments of non-fluency is not surprising. Differences among types of non-fluencies with equal severity, however, require explanation. At least one plausible explanation for the tendency to label sound and syllable repetitions as stuttering is available. If a judge intensionally defines stuttering as non-fluencies which involve difficulty in saying words, and regards non-fluencies involving difficulty in expressing ideas as normal, then it is plausible that he would associate sound and syllable repetitions with difficulty in saying a word rather than with difficulty in formulating an idea, and so would be more likely to classify this type of non-fluencies as stuttering. On the other hand, revisions and interjections could plausibly be associated with difficulty in expressing ideas and to the degree that this is

true they would not be labeled as stuttering.

It has been found that both adults and children who have been diagnosed as stutterers present proportionately more sound and syllable repetitions than do non-stutterers (1, 2, 3). Also, sound and syllable repetitions, according to the results of the present study, are relatively likely to be labeled 'stuttering.' The importance, however, of this labeling response in the original classification of individuals as stutterers is yet to be investigated. Three important questions have yet to be answered: (1) Are sound and syllable repetitions more or less likely to be labeled stuttering when they occur than when they do not occur in a context of meaningful connected speech? (2) Are perceived instances of non-fluency the chief determinant of the classification of a child as a stutterer? (3) Are there proportionately more sound and syllable repetitions in the speech of children classified as stutterers at the time when they are originally so classified than in the speech of children of comparable age and development who are not classified as stutterers? If all three of the above questions were to be answered in the affirmative, then the significance of sound and syllable repetitions in contributing to the classification of given speakers as stutterers would be established.

The results of this study confirm an earlier report by Tuthill (7) that judges trained in speech pathology do more labeling of speech phenomena as stuttering than do untrained judges. In the present study the judges knew when each example of non-fluency was to occur. Apparently the untrained judge, even when he is aware of a non-fluency, is less likely to label it as stuttering than the trained judge. Training in speech pathology as represented by the judges employed in this study, may thus not only increase awareness of non-fluencies, but it may also decrease tolerance for such speech phenomena.

Summary

Three groups of judges, two groups trained in speech pathology at two different institutions, respectively, and one group with no such training, classified each of 600 short speech samples as containing a stuttering non-fluency or as containing a non-stuttering non-fluency. Half of the speech samples were from the speech of stutterers and half were from the speech of non-stutterers. The samples had also been rated for severity of non-fluency by another group of listeners.

The frequency with which the judges applied the stuttering label varied with the rated severity of the samples. Trained judges applied the label more often than untrained judges. Sound and syllable repetitions were labeled as stuttering more often than revisions and interjections, regardless of rated severity. Judges, in general, agreed best on the severe stuttering non-fluencies and next best on the mild non-stuttering non-fluencies. The lowest agreement was on the severe non-stuttering non-fluencies and the next lowest on the mild stuttering non-fluencies.

Acknowledgement

Co-operation of Dr. Martin F. Palmer, Director of the Institute of Logopedics, is acknowledged gratefully.

References

1. CESARETTI, M.; A study of the nonfluency of first grade children. M.A. Thesis, Humboldt State College, 1958.

2. JOHNSON, W. (ed.), Analysis of recorded speech samples, Chapter 8, *The Onset of Stuttering*. Minneapolis: University of Minnesota Press, (in press).

3. JOHNSON, W., Normative studies of fluency. Unpublished research, University of Iowa.

4. JOHNSON, W., Studies in language behavior. I. A program of research. *Psychol. Monogr.*, 56, 1944, 1-15.

5. LINDQUIST, E. F., *Design and Analysis of Experiments in Psychology and Education*. Boston: Houghton Mifflin, 1953.

6. THURSTONE, L. L. and CHAVE, E. L., *The Measurement of Attitude*. Chicago: University of Chicago Press, 1929.

7. TUTHILL, C. E., A quantitative study of extensional meaning with special reference to stuttering. *Speech Monogr.*, 13, 1946, 81-98.

THE RELATION OF REPETITIONS IN THE SPEECH OF YOUNG CHILDREN TO CERTAIN MEASURES OF LANGUAGE MATURITY AND SITUATIONAL FACTORS: PART I[1]

DOROTHY M. DAVIS,
State University of Iowa,
Iowa City, Iowa

The occurrence and interpretation of repetitions in the speech of young children is not an entirely new problem to those interested in the development of language. Fröschels (3) has commented on repetitions, stating that it is not uncommon to find repetitions in infant speech, and that they are hardly pathological, but do lay, he feels, the groundwork for the pathological state if the child is embarrassed by his repetitions. Stinchfield (6) refers to them as slight signs of stuttering, occurring before the child has sufficient control of the speech mechanism to make it entirely automatic. Other statements have been made, such as those of Kirkpatrick (4) who believes that children repeat because they do not have tangible evidence that they have been understood. Interpretations put upon these repetitions obviously differ, and by differing raise the question of interpretative emphasis.

Some few studies have reported the extent of repetition, but usually "repetition" was considered as a self-explanatory term without a clear-cut definition of what was meant. Smith (5) reported the average number of repetitions per word used at each age level from the records of one hour of speech of each of eighty-eight children. Her results were:

Age, Years	Repetitions Divided by Number of Words Used
2	.114
3	.045
4	.022
5	.017

Fisher (2) took nine to twelve hours of stenographic records of the speech of seventy-two preschool children. She studied the amounts of repetition found, defining repetition as "exact repetition

---

[1]This study was done in the Iowa Child Welfare Research Station and the Speech Clinic, University of Iowa. It was directed by Wendell Johnson.

JOURNAL OF SPEECH DISORDERS, 1939, Vol. 4, pp. 303-318.

of the same remark, verbal or nonverbal with no variation in word or sound pattern." She found a correlation of —.73±.04 between chronological age and the per cent of exact repetition. She found that a large proportion of the repetition occurred in questions asked of adults, and stated that the unheeding adult puts the child under a repetitive compulsion. The boys were found to repeat more than the girls with 74 chances in 100 of there being a true difference.

None of the studies just mentioned have defined repetition by example, nor have any of them broken repetition into types such as syllable, word, or phrase repetition. There is no mention of normative amounts of repetition for different age-sex groups.

Egland (1) compared "stuttering" and "nonstuttering" children with respect to amounts of repetition through an ingenious puppet technique. This type of study raises the question of the reliability and validity of any criteria which might be used for separating "stutterers" from "nonstutterers."

For some time workers in the field of child psychology and speech pathology have thought that the discrimination of the "stuttering" and the "nonstuttering" child was relatively simple with listening to speech as the basis. Yet it is apparent that there never has been an objective, clear-cut definition of what constituted "stuttering." Unquestionably, every speaking adult and every speaking child at some times and in certain circumstances repeats himself. Many so-called young stutterers, who are not reacting to their speech emotionally merely present "normal" repetitions in their speech, for it is only after "psychological pressure" is put on them that facial grimaces, inhalatory difficulties, peculiar sounds, and "stallers" enter into the speech pattern as they apparently attempt to break or inhibit their repetitions. It would appear that before children are aware that parents or teachers consider their speech abnormal, repetitions are often not associated with other conspicuous types of interruptive speech phenomena. If, at an early age, the distinction between the pathological and the normal is one of quantity rather than quality, no attempts at separating "stutterers" from "nonstutterers" can be made without a measure of the amount of repetition found in the case of the average child. Such a measure would eliminate the careless labeling of a child a "stutterer" by parents and teachers merely on the basis of the presence of repetitions in his speech, thereby laying the stage for all of the unfortunate reactions which are often found associated with the speech of those who are unsure of their ability to speak acceptably.

As a first approach to this whole problem the following questions were formulated:

1. What is the nature of the distribution of repetitions in the speech of young children when repetitions are fractionated into syllable, word, and phrase repetitions?

2. What norms can be established for different age groups of boys and girls through the preschool years when the instances of

33

repetition and the total number of repetitive elements of syllable, word, and phrase repetition are considered?

3. Do any of the distributions show a measure which serves to segregate in a marked way the extremes from the bulk of the cases for possible purposes of diagnosis of fluency deficiencies?

4. For each age-sex group, what are the findings with regard to the average number of times each repetitive syllable, word, and phrase was repeated? What is the average length of repeated phrases?

5. Are there significant age-sex differences in any of these measures?

In order to attempt an answer to these questions the following research was undertaken.

The subjects used in the study were sixty-two children, thirty-six boys and twenty-six girls enrolled in the Preschool Laboratory of the Iowa Child Welfare Research Station. They ranged in age from twenty-four to sixty-two months, and the range in IQ's was from 105 to 162.

The data for this portion of the study were gathered by recording verbatim the speech of each child for an hour. The hour was broken into two half-hour periods and the records taken within one week of the day of the month corresponding to the birth date. The midpoint of the two days of recording was considered the date on which the data were gathered. All records were made during the free play period in the preschool routine when teacher-domination was at a minmum. The records were taken in a type of speed writing, devised by the experimenter, in order to keep pace with those children who talked very rapidly.

In the analysis, repetitions were considered a bit more broadly than in terms of exact duplications. The following presentation of the definitions and their qualifications will clarify what was meant:

1. A repetition is defined as the utterance of the same syllable, word, or group of words more than once. For example: "I want, I want to go."

2. The addition of "yes" or "no" to the repeated phrase does not vitiate the repetition. For example: "Put it in her wagon. No, put it in her wagon."

3. The addition of "too" or "hey" still preserves the repetition. For example: "Hey, here's some over here. Here's some over here too."

4. There can be repetition within a repetition which counts as a total of two repetitions. For example: "Put it in her wagon. Put it, put it, put it in her wagon."

5. A total response which is repeated at the beginning of the following response counts as a phrase repetition. For example: "You can't. You can't have any."

6. A phrase repetition may occur as part of one response, or involve the repetition of a total response. For example: "What are these things? What are these things?" or "What are these, what are these things?"
7. The calling of an individual's name over and over counts as a repetition. For example: "Mary. Mary. Mary."
8. The absence of the definite or the indefinite article does not vitiate the response as a repetition, because of the difficulty of detecting it in rapid speech. For example: "You sleep in the dog house You sleep in dog house."
9. Two complete responses can be repeated as a group, in which case they are scored as two repetitions. For example: "Oh, look what he's doing. He's putting his feet in the dog house. Oh, look what he's doing. He's putting his feet in the dog house."
10. The insertion of the name does not cancel the repetition. For example: "Let's rock on the rocking horse. Timmy, let's rock on the rocking horse."

The following limitations on repetitions were established:

1. Changes of one word essential to the meaning of the response nullify it as a repetition. For example: "That's all I need. That's all we need."
2. "What" or "hunh" when repeated were not scored as repetitions because their presence may be indicative of the child's inability to hear a remark made to him by another.
3. The insertion of a nonidentical remark between identical remarks cancels the repetition. For example: "We won't go down, will we? Watch. We won't go down, will we?"
4. Sounds made in imitation of motors, gas being put in a car, or water coming out of a hose, etc., were not scored as repetitions, since the child was attempting to imitate a continuous sound. For example: "Errrrrn. Errrrrrrn. Errrrrrn" (a motor).
5. A change of sentence structure nullifies the response. For example: "You can't. You cannot."

Unintelligible repeated syllables were included among the repetitions on the ground that they may have carried meaning to the child if not to the ear of the adult recorder.

Since the study concerned repetitions as a part of communicative speech, repetitions of either meaningful or nonsensical syllables, words, or phrases for the apparent enjoyment of rhythm were eliminated. The elimination was made on the basis of detection of rhythmical form in which the word or group of words repeated presented a chanting quality, a definite recurrence of pitch pattern, a regular cadence or emphasis.

With the concept of repetition determined, an analysis of the speech sample of each child was made in terms of the following twelve measures.

1. The instances of repeated words multiplied by the number of times each was repeated, added, plus the number of instances of syllable repetition, plus the number of words repeated in phrases multiplied by the number of times each was repeated, all divided by the number of words spoken.

2. The sum of the number of instances of syllable repetition was divided by the total number of words spoken.

3. The sum of the instances of word repetition was divided by the total number of words spoken.

4. The sum of the instances of phrase repetition was divided by the total number of words spoken.

5. The number of instances of word repetition plus the number of instances of phrase repetition was divided by the total number of words spoken.

6. The sum of the number of syllable, word, and phrase repetitions was divided by the total number of words spoken.

7. The instances of syllable repetition were multiplied by the number of times each syllable was repeated, added, and divided by the total number of words spoken.

8. The instances of word repetition were multiplied by the number of times each word was repeated, added, and divided by the total number of words spoken.

9. Phrase repetitions were treated by multiplying the number of words in each repetitive phrase by the number of times each was repeated, these values added, and the total divided by the number of words spoken.

10. Measures 8 and 9 were combined (as measures 3 and 4 were combined to give measure 5).

11. The average number of times syllables, words, and phrases were repeated was determined.

12. The average length of repeated phrases was computed.

The analysis yielded the following results:

The distribution of repetitions, scored in terms of the percentage of all words uttered, represented by those words repeated in part, in whole singly, and in whole in phrases, presented a fairly normal distribution. It is assumed that the apparent bimodality of the curve represents a sampling peculiarity, although the possibility of other interpretations is not to be overlooked. (See Figure 1.)

The mean of this distribution was 24.04 per cent and the standard deviation of the distribution 8.97 per cent. This distribution tended to show that repetition is not unique in a select group of children, but is part of the speech pattern of all children, as judged by the

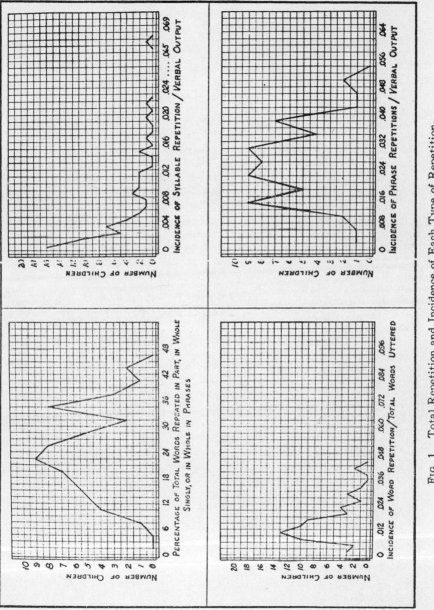

Fig. 1. Total Repetition and Incidence of Each Type of Repetition.

group here studied. It also shows that the amount of repetition varied from child to child, some repeating relatively less and others relatively more than the bulk of the group. All the children in the group repeated some words. The range of percentages ran from 6.2 per cent to 43.9 per cent of all words spoken. This material would tend to show that a child whose speech is such that approximately one word in four is a repeated word, either in part or in whole in a word or phrase repetition, is not presenting any abnormality in speech, but is talking "normally."

In consideration of the instances of syllable repetition in terms of verbal output a very different picture was presented. (See Figure 1.) The distribution showed extreme skewness to the right. The mean of the distribution was .004. Of the sixty-two children studied, sixteen did not present any syllable repetitions, and one child was 12.4 standard deviations beyond the mean, with 66 repetitions per thousand words. This child was the one child in the group studied who was judged a "stutterer" by parents and teachers alike.

It is interesting to note that the distribution did not extend unbrokenly from the mean to this point, but that for a distance of 8.8 standard deviations there was no child represented. It is unfortunate that there was not a larger group with more so-called "stutterers" in it, so that it might have been determined whether the distribution would have been continuous to this point or whether it would have been distinctly bimodal. The boy who scored 0.21, the highest scoring child on the main portion of the distribution, was considered a "stutterer" by one teacher, whereas several other teachers were concerned about his speech, but had not decided whether or not he "stuttered." (Since the completion of this study, the mother voluntarily brought this child to the Speech Clinic as a "stutterer.") The girl who scored .019, just two less syllable repetitions in a thousand words, had apparently attracted little attention to herself.

There were five children in this group who had been termed "stutterers" the year prior to the one in which this study was made. They scored as follows: 0, .003, .005, .009, .016. These scores would tend to show that either there was no diagnostic value in this scale, or that the children had been erroneously dubbed "stutterers" in the sense that they had never done an unusual amount of repeating, or that they had improved markedly in the intervening year. Although there are not data to substantiate any of these views, it is the writer's opinion that a combination of the last two possibilities accounted for the findings. It is perhaps possible that there was some basis for the concern over the child who scored .016, although it is to be emphasized that the question would have to be settled on the basis of various items of information in addition to this score of .016.

In consideration of the instances of whole word repetitions in terms of verbal output the distribution was found to be skewed to the right. (See Figure 1.) The mean of the distribution was .014, and the range was from 0 to .041. The child who scored .041 was the youngest child in the group studied. This distribution showed that

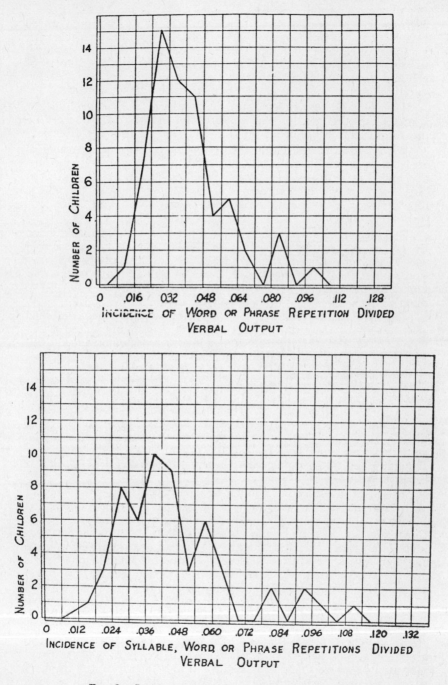

Fig. 2. Incidence of Types of Repetition Grouped.

the average child repeated fourteen words in every thousand words he spoke. Again there was individual variation on this measure with a number of children tending to repeat words more than the average, as was shown by the fact that there was little spread in the number of children repeating less than the mean amount, and considerable variation among those repeating more than the mean amount.

The so-called "stutterer" and the "possible stutterers" did not stand out on the basis of this measure, nor in any of the succeeding measures except those in relation to which they will be mentioned.

With regard to the instances of phrase repetitions in terms of verbal output the distribution was found to be roughly symmetrical and approximately normal. (See Figure 1.) The mean of the distribution was .025, which means that the average number of phrase repetitions in a thousand words was twenty-five. The range was from .010 to .048.

The incidence of word and phrase repetitions totaled and divided by the verbal output presented a distribution that was skewed toward the high values. (See Figure 2.) The mean of the distribution was .041, and the range was .015 to .097. The child who repeated ninety-seven times in a thousand words was a girl of twenty-five months.

The instances of syllable, word, and phrase repetitions combined and divided by the total number of words spoken presented a distribution skewed toward the higher number of repetitions. (See Figure 2.) The mean of the distribution was .045, and the range was from .017 to .113. The child who repeated 113 times in a thousand words was the so-called "stutterer." Although he here received the highest score, it should be noted that he did not appear to deviate so markedly as when syllable repetitions alone were considered. Since he did not show marked deviation in any measures except those dealing with syllable repetition, combination measures which included word or phrase repetitions tended to pull him closer to the balance of the group and to camouflage his deviation in the measure of syllable repetitions.

The distribution of the number of repetitive syllables in terms of verbal output (that is, the instances of syllable repetition, multiplied by the number of times each syllable was repeated, and the sum of these values divided by the number of words spoken) was an exceedingly interesting one. (See Figure 3.) It was markedly skewed to the high scores. Sixteen children presented no syllable repetitions and twenty-eight had less than five in a thousand words. The mean of the distribution was .013, showing that the average child used thirteen syllable repetitions in a thousand words. The range in scores was from zero to .168. The child who used 168 repetitive syllables in one thousand words was the so-called "stutterer." This child was found to be 8.8 standard deviations from the mean of the group. The child next to him, who scored .076, was the boy of forty-nine months whose speech was beginning to be noted by the teachers as dangerously approaching "stuttering." In this measure was

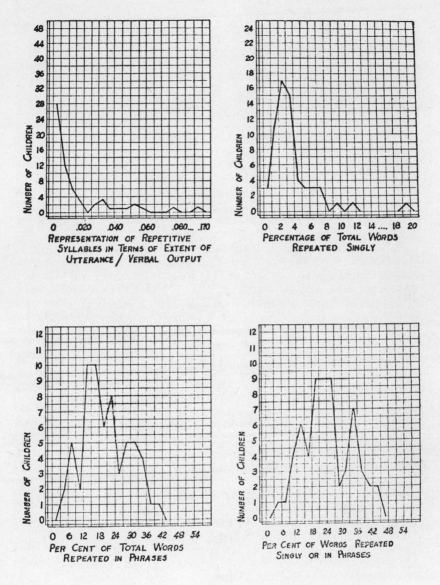

Fig. 3.

41

found the possibility of segregating extremes from the balance of the group.

The distribution of the percentage of words used in a repetitive fashion was also skewed, but not so much as the measure of repetitive syllables. (See Figure 3.) The mean of the distribution was 3.6 per cent, and the range was from zero to 19 per cent. The two who ranked highest with 19 and 11.4 per cent were the two youngest girls studied.

The percentage of words used in repetivite phrases was somewhat skewed, but less than either the use of repetitive syllables or repetitive words. (See Figure 3.) The mean of the distribution was 20.4 per cent and the range was from 3.2 to 40.9 per cent. The child who used 40.9 words in repetitive phrases in one hundred words was the boy of thirty-nine months who rated highest in the first measure, the composite measure. He was not regarded by anyone as a 'stutterer.''

The distribution of the percentage of words used repetitively in both word and phrase repetitions combined presented a more nearly normal distribution. (See Figure 3.) The mean of this distribution was 24 per cent, and the range was from 3.5 to 43 9 per cent.

In consideration of all of these measures it was found that the two which deal with the instances of syllable repetition and with the number of repetitive syllables used in syllable repetitions, were the best measures for determining the children who deviated markedly from the group. In each of these measures the child who was termed a "stutterer" stands out dramatically from the balance of the group. The percentage of repetitive words out of the total number of words used is probably the next best single measure, but it tended to segregate three children, two of whom were the two youngest girls in the group studied. This would lead to the tentative conclusion that this measure was penalizing the younger children and not segregating the children of all ages who deviated markedly.

The attention of those concerned with the evaluation of repetitions in the speech of young children for the purposes of determining marked deviation from the group should be directed to a study of the child's syllable repetitions.

The distribution of the average number of times repetitive syllables were repeated was a skewed distribution (See Figure 4.) The low values were the range in which the majority of cases fell. The mean of the distribution was 2.25. Sixteen children did not repeat any syllables, so that their scores were zero this measure. There could not be values between zero and two because of the nature of repetitions. By "two" is meant that the syllable was said twice, not repeated twice. Fourteen children had a mean of two. The highest mean score on this measure was 4.39, scored by the boy of forty-three months, a "nonstutterer," who scored highest on the composite measure and on the percentage of words used in repetitive phrases.

The distribution of the mean number of times repetitive words were said did not show a great amount of spread. (See Figure 4.)

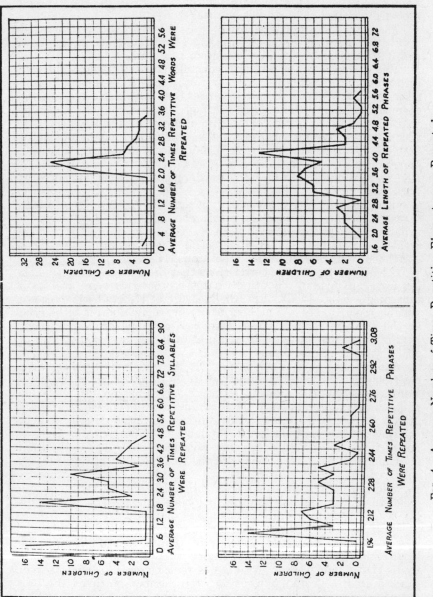

FIG. 4. Average Number of Times Repetitive Elements were Repeated.

43

There was only one child, a girl of twenty-nine months, who repeated no words. The other children in the group clustered between 2 and 3.3.

The mean number of times each repetitive phrase was said showed more scatter than either of the other two means. (See Figure 4.) The mean of the distribution was 2.25. All the children repeated phrases; the highest score was 3.

The mean length of repeated phrases showed a distribution that approached normalcy. (See Figure 4.). The mean of the distribution was 3.67 words, and the range was from 2.0 to 5.5.

The question of whether those children who ranked high in instances of either syllable, word, or phrase repetition ranked high in either or both of the other two measures is an important one. If the correlations among these three are high, then it can be concluded that any single one is a good measure of repetitions as a whole. The correlation of the instances of syllable repetition with the instances of word repetition was $.40 \pm .11$. The instances of syllable repetition correlated with the instances of phrase repetition was $.09 \pm .13$. The correlation of instances of word repetition with instances of phrase repetition was $.34 \pm .11$.

In correlating the total extent of syllable repetitions with the extent of word repetitions the result was $.35 \pm .11$. The extent of syllable repetitions correlated with the extent of phrase repetitions yielded a coefficient of $.03 \pm .13$. The extent of word repetitions correlated with that of phrase repetitions $.11 \pm .13$.

It is shown from these correlations that the possibility of predicting from one type of repetition what the other two types will be is exceedingly limited. If, then, the measure of either the instance of syllable repetition or the number of repetitive syllables is to be used as the measure for separating extremes from the group, it is not justifiable to substitute for it measures of the extent or instances of either word or phrase repetitions.

Another question which should be answered is whether those children who present the largest number of instances of syllable, word, or phrase repetitions in terms of verbal output are the same children who rank highest in the total amounts of syllable, word, and phrase repetition, respectively, determined in terms of extent.

The correlation of instances of syllable repetition with total number of repetitive syllable elements was $.96 \pm .01$. The correlation of instances of word repetition with the total number of single words used repetitively was $.97 \pm .008$. These two correlations show a high degree of agreement in that the children who had the high incidence of syllable and word repetition also presented a large number of repetitive words and syllables, respectively.

With regard to phrases the findings were somewhat different. The correlation between incidence of phrase repetitions and the length and extent of phrase repetitions was $.67 \pm .07$. This finding shows that there was no great agreement between the number of times a child repeated phrases and the number of times the repetitive phrases were repeated by him.

In addition, the data show that the children in this study used more phrase repetitions than word or syllable repetitions, and more word repetitions than syllable repetitions. This is in keeping with the finding that syllable repetitions are more diagnostic of extreme amounts of repetition, for the more frequent an occurrence, the less unusual it is.

For the purpose of deriving norms the group was divided into three age levels, with the boys separated from the girls. The three age levels were: twenty-four to thirty-five months; thirty-six to forty-nine months; and fifty to sixty months. Medians were derived for each group and the results are given in Table 1.

It will be noted that there are differences in the various measures from age-group to age-group, and that the boys and the girls do not have identical medians. In order to determine what age-sex differences were obtained, critical ratios were computed. From these ratios the following conclusions were derived.

TABLE I

MEDIAN VALUES FOR CHRONOLOGICAL AGE GROUPS, MEASURES OF SYLLABLE, WORD, AND PHRASE REPETITIONS

	AGE MONTHS			
	24 to 35	36 to 49	50 to 60	Total
	GIRLS			
	8	7	11	26
Composite measure................	.348	.266	.157	.241
Instances of syllable repetition divided by verbal output..........	0	.003	.001	.001
Instances of word repetition divided by verbal output.................	.011	.011	.009	.009
Instances of phrase repetition divided by verbal output.................	.031	.027	.018	.023
Instances of word and phrase repetitions divided by verbal output....	.041	.042	.027	.034
Instances of syllable, word, and phrase repetitions divided by verbal output	.041	.046	.026	.034
Number of repetitive syllables divided by verbal output..........	0	.0068	.0033	.0033
Number of repetitive words divided by verbal output.................	1.7 per cent	2.6 per cent	1.9 per cent	2.0 per cent
Number of repetitive words used in repetitive phrases divided by verbal output...........................	28 per cent	22.7 per cent	13.9 per cent	20.5 per cent
Number of repetitive words used in repetitive words and phrases divided by verbal output..........	34.8 per cent	25.8 per cent	15.3 per cent	23.9 per cent
Mean number of times repetitive syllables were repeated..........	0	2.67	2.00	2.00
Mean number of times repetitive words were repeated..............	2.14	2.25	2.25	2.25
Mean number of times repetitive phrases were repeated.............	2.35	2.20	2.18	2.20
Mean length of repetitive phrases....	3.90	3.51	3.75	3.73

TABLE I—(Continued)

	Age, Months			
	24 to 35	36 to 49	50 to 60	Total
	Boys			
	7	13	16	36
Composite measure..................	.297	.239	.219	.229
Instances of syllable repetition divided by verbal output..........	.004	.001	.004	.003
Instances of word repetition divided by verbal output..................	.021	.013	.012	.013
Instances of phrase repetition divided by verbal output..................	.036	.025	.024	.025
Instances of word and phrase repetitions divided by verbal output....	.057	.037	.039	.038
Instances of syllable, word, and phrase repetitions divided by verbal output	.063	.039	.042	.045
Number of repetitive syllables divided by verbal output..........	.0089	.0056	.0125	.0085
Number of repetitive words divided by verbal output..................	4.8 per cent	3.0 per cent	2.8 per cent	3.0 per cent
Number of repetitive words used in repetitive phrases divided by verbal output.....................	20.4 per cent	20.6 per cent	17.4 per cent	18.9 per cent
Number of repetitive words used in repetitive words and phrases divided by verbal output..........	26.7 per cent	23.6 per cent	21.3 per cent	23.2 per cent
Mean number of times repetitive syllables were repeated...........	2.00	2.00	2.89	2.61
Mean number of times repetitive words were repeated..............	2.29	2.27	2.43	2.29
Mean number of times repetitive phrases were repeated.............	2.15	2.14	2.12	2.14
Mean length of repetitive phrases....	3.78	4.00	3.52	3.68

With respect to age differences, viewing all of the measures for both boys and girls, the general trend, with the exception of the measures where syllable repetitions alone were considered, was in the direction of a decrease in amount with age. As a rule, however, this trend was completely significant only when the lowest age-group was compared with either of the other older age-groups. These findings indicate that if there are true age differences, they are probably confined to the comparison of the two younger age-groups.

With respect to sex differences, these data showed the most striking differences in the instances of syllable repetition and the extent of syllable repetition. These differences, as a rule, favored the boys (i. e., showed that the boys repeated more). Other measures did not show clear-cut sex differences.

Summary

In a study of one hour of the extemporaneous speech of each of 62 children ranging in age from twenty-four to sixty-two months, it was found that repetitions, when those involving syllables, words, and phrases were combined, showed a fairly normal distribution with all the children in the group represented. Even though the amount of repetition varied from child to child, it was concluded that repetition is part of the speech pattern of all children. The distribution of syllable repetition showed extreme skewness to the right, and it is unfortunate that there were not more so-called "stutterers" in the group to serve as subjects in the testing of the clinical validity of this finding. Both instances of syllable repetition and the number of repetitive syllables used in syllable repetitions were found to be the best measures for determining those children who deviated markedly from the group.

With respect to the extent of syllable, word, and phrase repetitions, averages are given. Prediction from the extent of one type of repetition to another is exceedingly limited. Those children who had a high incidence of syllable and word repetition also presented a large number of repetitive words and syllables, respectively; but there was no great agreement between the number of times a child repeated phrases and the number of times the repetitive phrases were repeated by him. In order of frequency of occurrence, the types of repetition ranked: phrase, word, syllable.

The children were divided into three age groups and the boys and girls separated. Medians for each group were obtained and are presented in Table I. Although there appears to be a decrease with age in amounts of repetition, it would appear that true differences are confined to a comparison of the younger two age groups. Syllable repetition appears unaffected by age within the limits of the population examined.

No clear-cut sex differences were observable with the exception of measures dealing with syllable repetition. These measures indicated more repetition for boys than for girls.

REFERENCES

1. **Egland, George O.** An analysis of repetition and prolongations in the speech of young children. State University of Iowa, Unpublished Master's thesis, 1938.
2. **Fisher, Mary Shattuck.** Language patterns of preschool children. J. Exper. Educ., 1932–1933, 1, 70–85.
3. **Froeschels, Emil.** Psychological elements in speech . . . in company with Professor Ottmar Dittrick and Frau Dr. Ilka Wilhelm. Trans. by Nils Ferre. Boston, Mass. Expression Co., (c. 1932) Pp. xvii, 270.
4. **Kirkpatrick, E. A.** How children learn to talk. Science, 1891, 18, 175. Cited by Brandenburg, George C.: The Language of a Three-Year-Old Child. Ped. Sem., 1915, 22, 89–120.
5. **Smith, Madorah Elizabeth.** An investigation of the development of the sentence and the extent of vocabulary in young children. Univ. Iowa Stud., Stud. in Child Welfare, 1926, 3, No. 5, Pp. 92.
6. **Stinchfield, Sarah M.** A preliminary study in corrective speech. Univ. Iowa Stud., Stud. in Child Welfare, 1930, 1, No. 3, Pp. 36.

THE RELATION OF REPETITIONS IN THE SPEECH OF YOUNG CHILDREN TO CERTAIN MEASURES OF LANGUAGE MATURITY AND SITUATIONAL FACTORS

Part II*

Dorothy M. Davis, Ph. D.

Indiana State Teachers College,
Terre Haute, Indiana

Part I of this series of articles dealt with repetitions of syllables, words, and phrases in the speech of preschool children observed during free play. The second portion of this research concerns some of the factors which may superficially appear to be instrumental in the development of the phenomenon of repetition, namely language development. Adams (1) approached the problem of relating repetitions to measures of language growth, but he did not fractionate repetitions, nor did he draw any direct comparisons between repetitions and language growth. Consequently, his study is suggestive but does not answer the question of relationship conclusively.

Language maturity is a term which needs further delineation in this report. In this study it refers to measures of vocabulary extent, percentage of incomplete responses, percentage of simple responses, percentage of complete responses, number of speech sounds correctly articulated, length of response, percentage of functionally complete responses, and the proportion of intelligible responses.

Samples of speech for each of sixty-two preschool children between the ages of two and five years were collected in two half-hour periods chosen from the free-play portion of the preschool routine. This material furnished the basis for the structural analysis of each child's speech. The first step in the analysis was the determination of the limits of each response and the establishment of the mean length of response for each child. A response was considered to be a speech unit which was either a complete sentence or a portion of a sentence if the latter was set off by pauses. The pauses were noted while the recording was being done.

The counting of words for the establishment of the mean length of response offered some problems. The criteria used by McCarthy (2) were a guide.

1. Contractions of a noun or pronoun and a verb were considered as two words because both are essential to the response if it is to be considered grammatically complete.

---

*This study was done in the Iowa Child Welfare Research Station and the Speech Clinic, University of Iowa. It was directed by Wendell Johnson.

JOURNAL OF SPEECH DISORDERS, 1940, Vol. 5
pp. 235-241.

2. Contractions of a verb form and "not," such as "won't" and "can't" were scored as one word. Since the child presumably has little knowledge of reading and writing, he probably thinks of "can" and "can't" as the two possibilities in expression. If he uses "cannot" it is highly improbable that he associates it with the contracted form "can't."

3. "Lookit" was scored as one word if it served in the capacity of "look," and as two words if it served as "look at."

4. Hyphenated words which must occur together to convey thought were scored as one word, such as "teeter-totter."

5. Nonsense syllables were arbitrarily counted as words. With nonsense it is impossible to discern the limits of the pseudo-words, so some arbitrary practice had to be instituted.

6. After the establishment of word limits, the total number of words spoken in the entire hour was counted for each child. This is referred to in this report as the "verbal output."

The speech records were also analyzed for indices of language maturity. The degree of intelligibility was considered one gauge of maturity. Since understandability of language is essential to its communicative effectiveness, the degree of comprehensibility is an index to the facility with which it is used in communication. McCarthy's (2, p. 35) criteria of intelligibility were adopted. Three classifications were used, as described below:

1. "Comprehensible responses which included all responses that could be understood by the experimenter in spite of poor articulation, letter substitutions, or faulty or incomplete construction.

2. "Semi-comprehensible responses which included all responses in which the hearer (recorder) had a general idea of what the child was talking about, but could not get the full meaning because of the lack of certain key words in the sentence.

3. "Incomprehensible vocalizations which included all responses which were mere sounds forming no recognizable words, and which were entirely devoid of meaning to the hearer."

The McCarthy classification of grammatical complexity was used with one adaptation. First of all, responses were divided into two main groups: those that were complete and those that were incomplete. In a consideration of spoken language, we are impressed with the fact that much of adult language is fragmentary. Conversation among adults carries a multiplicity of responses in which a number of the elements of the sentence are omitted. Such responses as "all right," "fine," and "good" have neither subject nor predicate, and so cannot be considered a sentence, but the assumptions of the noun and verb are clear, and the response is adequate for communication. Because the child learns the language patterns which he hears, his speech should be judged in terms of a standard no more severe than that used for the evaluation of adult speech. Therefore, fragmentary responses of the sort discussed above were termed "functionally complete but structurally incomplete responses."

The following classification was used in the structural analysis of the responses:

A. Complete responses.
1. Functionally complete but structurally incomplete responses.
2. Simple sentences without a prepositional phrase.
3. Simple sentences with a prepositional phrase.
4. Compound sentences.
5. Complex sentences.
6. Compound-complex sentences.

B. Incomplete responses.
C. Incomprehensible responses not analyzed structurally.

In this study, the functionally complete but structurally incomplete responses were treated as a unit, and the proportion of the total number of responses that this type represented was determined. Simple sentences both with and without prepositional phrases were combined to form the measure of simple responses. Compound, complex, and compound-complex responses were grouped to represent a measure of complex responses. The proportion of incomplete responses was also determined. These, then, were the measures of language maturity used in this study to represent complexity of response structure.

In the analyses described above repetitions of phrases were omitted from consideration, for in the case of whole response repetitions the saying of the response more than once would tend to weight the frequency of that grammatical construction on which the repetition occurred.

Vocabulary was tested by means of the Smith-Williams Vocabulary Test (3).

Speech sounds were tested on the Williams revision of the Wellman, Case, Mengert, and Bradbury Speech Sounds Test (4). This test was chosen because of the ease of administration and the clarity with which it detects speech sound errors.

Other tests of general maturity which were used included chronological age, mental age, and the intelligence quotient as determined by the Kuhlmann-Binet or the Stanford-Binet tests.

Five of the measures representative of repetition were correlated with the various measures of language maturity and general development. The measures of repetition chosen were the composite measure, instances of syllable repetition, instances of word repetition, instances of phrase repetition, and the sum of the instances of syllable, word, and phrase repetitions. (See Part I) Correlations of the Pearson product-moment type were determined for all of these measures, and the following results obtained:

TABLE I

Correlation of Various Measures of General Development and Language Maturity with Five Measures of Repetition

	Composite Measure			Syllable Repetition/ Verbal Output			Word Repetition/ Verbal Output			Phrase Repetition/ Verbal Output			All Repetitions/ Verbal Output		
	Cases	r	S.E.	Cases	r	S.E.	Cases	r	S.E.	Cases	r	S.E.	Cases	r	S.E.
Chronological Age	62	−.48	.098	61	.05	.128	61	−.30	.116	62	−.37	.110	62	−.48	.098
Mental Age	55	−.44	.109	54	.05	.136	54	−.35	.119	55	−.29	.123	55	−.46	.106
Intelligence Quotient	55	−.05	.134	54	−.04	.136	54	−.10	.135	55	−.04	.135	55	.03	.135
Verbal Output	62	−.08	.126	61	−.01	.128	61	−.27	.119	62	−.07	.126	62	−.30	.116
Mean Length of Response	62	−.38	.109	61	.04	.128	61	−.47	.101	62	−.33	.113	62	−.56	.087
Vocabulary	59	−.47	.101	58	.13	.129	58	−.27	.122	59	−.35	.114	59	−.46	.103
Number Correct Speech Sounds	61	−.53	.092	60	.08	.128	60	−.19	.124	61	−.47	.100	61	−.37	.111
Per Cent Intelligibility	62	−.23	.120	61	.12	.126	61	−.37	.111	62	−.28	.117	62	−.32	.114
Per Cent Incomplete Responses	61	.33	.114	60	−.009	.129	61	.17	.124	61	.25	.120	61	.21	.122
Per Cent Functionally Complete Responses	62	.17	.123	61	.20	.123	61	.34	.113	62	.13	.125	62	.39	.108
Per Cent Simple Responses	62	−.19	.122	61	.004	.128	61	−.47	.100	62	−.15	.124	62	−.47	.099
Per Cent Complex Responses	62	−.41	.106	61	.07	.127	61	−.30	.116	62	−.35	.111	62	−.42	.105

A consideration of these correlations leads to the following conclusions:

1. None of these correlations is sufficiently large to be considered the key to an explanation of repetitions. The largest is the correlation of —.56 between syllable, word and phrase repetitions divided by verbal output and mean length of response, and even this correlation can be considered indicative of little more than a trend.

2. Chronological age showed correlations of approximately the same magnitude with each of these measures except syllable repetition divided by verbal output. This would indicate that there was a tendency toward a decrease in repetition with age with the possible exception of syllable repetitions where it may be concluded that there was no relationship.

3. Mental age showed a slight negative relationship to all measures of repetition divided by verbal output, tending to indicate that with the exception of syllable repetition where no relationship was present, there was a slight tendency for repetition to decrease with increased mental age.

4. I. Q. showed low correlations with all measures; it can be concluded that there was no relationship present.

5. Verbal output showed no particular relationship except with word repetition divided by verbal output and instances of syllable, word and phrase repetitions divided by verbal output where there was a slight negative relationship.

6. Vocabulary showed a low correlation with negative direction with all measures of repetition except syllable repetition with which no relation was shown.

7. Correct articulation showed a low negative correlation with the measures of repetition except syllable repetition.

8. The degree of intelligibility showed a negative correlation with the measures of repetition except syllable repetition.

9. The percentage of incomplete responses had a slight positive correlation with measures of repetition except syllable repetition.

10. The percentage of functionally complete but structurally incomplete responses had a slight positive correlation with all measures of repetition.

11. The correlations with percentage of simple responses were all low and negative with the exception of syllable repetitions which was practically zero.

12. Complex responses correlated low negatively with measures of repetition, except for syllable repetitions in which the correlation was almost zero.

13. It would appear that the incidence of syllable repetition was not significantly related to any of these measures.

Because it has already been established that vocabulary, mean length of responses, number of correct speech sounds, intelligibility, and percentage of complex responses are related to chronological age; chronological age was held constant and the partial correlations presented in Table II were computed.

TABLE II
PARTIAL CORRELATIONS WITH CHRONOLOGICAL AGE CONSTANT

	Composite Measure of Repetition	Syllable Repetition/ Verbal Output	Word Repetition/ Verbal Output	Phrase Repetition/ Verbal Output	All Repetitions/ Verbal Output
Mental Age	—.020	—.011	—.192	.106	—.073
Verbal Output	.234	—.043	—.137	.160	—.061
Mean Length of Response	—.049	.005	—.370	—.094	—.350
Vocabulary	—.107	.188	—.007	—.049	—.060
No. Correct Speech Sounds	—.462	.063	.007	—.325	—.087
Per Cent Intelligibility	.123	.115	—.241	—.056	—.012
Per Cent Incomplete Responses	.129	.017	.031	.089	—.026
Per Cent Functionally Complete Responses	.102	.212	.307	.073	.357
Per Cent Simple Responses	.108	—.029	—.382	.074	—.277
Per Cent Complex Responses	—.106	.049	—.127	—.130	—.122

Since mental age correlated .90 with chronological age, when chronological age is held constant in partial correlations, the correlations are also indicative of what would be found if mental age were held constant.

Because the instances of syllable repetition involved a noticeable sex difference at the various age levels studied, the boys and girls were separated and their scores on instances of syllable repetition were correlated with these various measures of maturity.

TABLE III
SYLLABLE REPETITIONS DIVIDED BY VERBAL OUTPUT

	Girls	r	Boys	r
Chronological Age	26	—.04	35	.05
Mental Age	23	.002	31	.04
Intelligence Quotient	23	.23	31	—.20
Verbal Output	25	.17	35	—.28
Vocabulary	25	.21	35	.03
Number Correct Speech Sounds	25	.02	33	.05
Per Cent Intelligibility	26	.14	35	.08
Per Cent Incomplete Responses	25	—.05	35	.01
Per Cent Functionally Complete Responses	26	.05	35	.32
Per Cent Simple Responses	26	.11	35	—.14
Per Cent Complex Responses	26	.06	35	.02

Summary and Conclusions

In this study an attempt was made to relate syllable, word, and phrase repetitions to various measures of language maturity. The data were obtained by recording verbatim the speech of sixty-two preschool children for a period of one hour chosen from the free-play portion of the preschool day. The repetitions found in this sample of speech were related by the correlation technique to measures of language complexity derived from the same speech sample.

From these measures of relationship it was concluded that language maturity as measured in this study cannot be considered an important factor in relation to repetition. When chronological age was held constant, the correlations tended to become even lower, although the relation to chronological age itself was not marked. To say that chronological age is important to a certain degree has no meaning, for in all probability it is not mere age that exerts the influence, but some as yet not uncovered factor of maturity which correlates with age. Correlations of syllable repetition alone and the measures of language maturity with boys and girls separated gave relationships which were almost insignificant.

From these findings it may be concluded tentatively that if it is desired to find the explanation for the large number of repetitions found in the speech of preschool children (see Part I) it must be sought elsewhere than in the area of language maturity, that is, that the child repeats because he is not adept at using language in the conventional manner.

REFERENCES

(1) **Adams, Sidney.** A study of the growth of language between two and four years. J. Juvenile Res., 1932, 16, 269–277.

(2) **McCarthy, Dorothea A.** The language development of the preschool child. University of Minnesota, Institute of Child Welfare Monog. Ser., No. 4. Minneapolis, Minnesota: University of Minnesota Press, 1930. Pp. xiii, 174.

(3) **Williams, Harold M.,** and **McFarland, Mary L.** A revision of the Smith vocabulary test for preschool children. (In) Williams, Harold M., McFarland, Mary L., and Little, Marguerite F., Development of Language and Vocabulary in Young Children. Univ. Iowa Stud., Stud. in Child Welfare, 1937, 13, No. 2, Pp. 94. (pp. 47–94).

(4) **Williams, Harold M.** An analytical study of language achievement in preschool children. (In) Williams, Harold M., McFarland, Mary L., and Little, Marguerite F., Development of Language and Vocabulary in Young Children. Univ. Iowa Stud., Stud. in Child Welfare, 1937, 13, No. 2, Pp. 94. (pp. 9–18).

THE RELATION OF REPETITIONS IN THE SPEECH OF YOUNG CHILDREN TO CERTAIN MEASURES OF LANGUAGE MATURITY AND SITUATIONAL FACTORS

Part III

Dorothy M. Davis, Ph. D.

Indiana State Teachers College,
Terre Haute, Indiana

It seems a fair assumption that many repetitions in speech may be associated in some manner with the semantic reactions of the speaker to the situations in which he finds himself. Case histories and reports of interviews obtained in the Speech Clinic of the State University of Iowa show that parents and guardians of repeating children believe that the child repeats relatively more in certain definite situations. These situations, as reported, show variation from child to child. Frequently mentioned in this connection are situations involving "fear," "excitement," "anger," and "thwarting." Since the so-called "stuttering child" does not live in a vacuum, but is reacting to the social stimuli about him, it cannot be said categorically that the given speech reactions which he exhibits are "abnormal." It is not known to what degree the so-called "normal speaking child," when placed in the same circumstances with the same semantic reactions to them, would or could retain nonrepetitive speech.

The problem in this portion of the study was to attempt an answer to the question of how extreme magnitudes of repetition relate to situational factors.

The technique used to furnish data for the approach to this problem was the observation of sixty-two children of preschool age. One recorder wrote verbatim all that was said by one child during two half-hour periods of observation during the free-play period in the preschool routine. Another observer was present who recorded as much as was possible of all that was said to the child and also the activity of the child and his companions. The second observer was asked not to interpret the situations, but to keep the record as nearly

JOURNAL OF SPEECH DISORDERS, 1940, Vol.5, pp.242-246.

as possible on the descriptive level. He was cautioned to be most explicit in describing the situations surrounding the appearance of repetitions. The influence of the two recorders on the child's speech can best be gauged by the reactions of the children. Both recorders attempted to keep in the background, avoiding a marked scrutiny of the child under observation while close to him. It was felt that neither observer was accepted in the same status as the preschool teachers, but rather as part of the furnishings. All conversation with the recorders was discouraged. It is thought that the recording attracted very little attention, for on only three occasions was any direct mention made of the process, and in only one of these did the child imply by his remarks that he thought that he was being watched.

The method of analysis of the data for repetitions was described in Part I of these articles: In connection with the situational analysis it was hoped to ascertain whether or not each repetition would be found accompanied by some recognizable factor or factors in the environment or situation which might succinctly account for its occurrence at that precise moment, and not at other moments chosen at random in the hour studied. This plan was abandoned because of the difficulty of discovering such factors. At this point there seemed such a superfluity of situations surrounding the repetition that no selective situations seemed to be present. This was true for one of two reasons: either there is no systematic situational tie-up for all repetitions or else the data on situations were too meager to reveal it.

It was observed, though, that in relation to extremes of repetition, those instances when a child uttered the same syllable, word, or phrase three or more times, certain situational factors could be recognized. Whether this is indicative of the true state of affairs surrounding repetitions, or whether it is the result of more care on the part of the recorder of situations in the presence of more extremes of repetition is a moot question.

An attempt was made to discover whether there were any types of classification that would include all the situations which appeared to foster extremes of repetition. Such a classification was developed in the following manner: Each extreme repetition was studied and an abbreviated description made of the activity accompanying it. From these descriptions the classification was built by a certain amount of grouping. Of course systematic measurement of the psychological forces at play in any of these situations was not feasible, so the classification was kept as nearly descriptive as possible. It should be remembered that these situations are *accompaniments* of repetition and also that each situation is discrete, grouping being used only in the hope of showing general tendencies. The writer is aware that these situations which are classified under any one grouping are not equal semantically (situation$_1$ $\neq$ situation$_2$ $\neq$ situation$_3$), and it is intended that the reader will evaluate any such groupings of situations accordingly, cognizant of the difficulties encountered in any such attempt at classification.

Before giving the situational findings it is well to have some conception of the proportion of all repetitions which the group studied included. It was found that 53.8 per cent of all syllable repetitions, 23.9 per cent of all word repetitions, and 15.6 per cent of all phrase repetitions were two or more in extent. It is interesting

.to note that syllable repetitions, which are conspicuous in every portion of the study, stand out here also as the measure in which more than half of the instances fall in what might be termed the "extreme extent range." Furthermore, it was found that thirty children presented no syllable repetitions two or more in extent, while eleven children presented only this type of syllable repetition. Nine children showed no extreme word repetitions whereas the balance of the group clustered around twenty-five per cent as a peak with the scores of ten children falling there. Extremes of phrase repetition skewed toward the higher percentages with thirteen children showing no phrase repetitions of this type, and only one child rated as high as fifty per cent. None of these three distributions could be considered "normal."

With phrases there was a clustering about the low end of the scale, and with both syllable and word repetition there was a clustering at two points, which was most marked in the case of syllable repetition.

The classification which was developed was as follows:

The child:

    wants an object possessed by another child.
    wants to perform an activity in which another child is engaged.
    tries to attract attention of teacher.
    tries to attract attention of child.
    wants to direct activity of teacher.
    wants to direct activity of child according to own plan.
    wants to direct child out of play group.
    asks teacher for information.
    asks teacher for object.
    asks teacher for privilege.
    shows excitement over own activity.
    receives coercion from teacher with object taken.
    receives coercion from teacher with activity changed.
    receives coercion from child with object taken.
    receives coercion from child with activity changed.
    offers criticism of child or his activity.
    boasts to teacher.
    boasts to child.
    shows surprise or astonishment at a child's possession.
    shows surprise or astonishment at a child's activity.
    upholds status in spite of another child.
    describes an object or activity to another.
    offers information to the teacher.
    offers information to child.
    appears to be trying for social acceptance or approbation.
    reports misconduct of a child to teacher.
    appears unable to think of next word or idea.
    defies the teacher.
    appears unable to find an object he searches.
    appears unable to find an individual he searches.
    is afraid or in pain.
    miscellaneous.

With respect to the order of rankings of the various situations, when the instances of all types of repetitions for all age-sex groups were combined, the following presented themselves as outstanding:

Rank	Item
1	excitement over own activity.
2	wants to direct activity of another child according to his own plan.
3	attempts to attract attention of child.
4	coerced by teacher resulting in changed activity.
5.5	attempts to attract attention of teacher.
5.5	upholds status in spite of another child.
7	offers information to another child.
8	wants an object possessed by another child.
9	criticizes another child.
10	offers information to teacher.

When the rankings were based on instances of syllable repetition alone the order was as follows:

Rank	Item
1	wants to direct activity of another child according to his own plan.
2	excitement over own activity.
3	coerced by teacher resulting in changed activity.
4	wants an object possessed by another child.
5.5	upholds status in spite of another child.
5.5	offers information to teacher.
7.5	offers information to child.
7.5	asks another child for information.
9.5	attempts to direct activity of teacher.
9.5	attempts to attract attention of teacher.

Word and phrase rankings were similar. Rankings based on the number of children represented in relation to instances of repetitions, and the mean percentage of each child's repetitions for syllables, words, and phrases for each situation in each age group show very similar rankings to these mentioned above.

The conclusions to be drawn from this study may be summarized, if we wish to consider the subjects used here as an adequate sample, as showing that all children in the age range of from two to five years repeat. Indeed, that though the amount of repetition differs from child to child, repetition is part of the speech pattern of all children. Repetitions of words and phrases decrease with age if the ages compared are far enough apart, but syllable repetition appears to be only slightly affected by age changes within this range. From the second portion of the study it was found that language maturity as defined herein relates only slightly to any of the types of repetition. The next area of inquiry is that which pertains to the situations themselves. It would be fruitful from the preventive standpoint if factors relating to repetitions could be found. Most studies dealing with so-called "stuttering" have been carried on with adults or near-adults, and there may be helpful material at hand if attention is given to those potential "stutterers," or individuals who may later attach pathological significance to their repetitions. It is of course trite to state that something acts as the adequate stimulus for repetitions. Repetitions in speech do not occur rhythmically. For some reason or reasons a child repeats at one particular instance and not at another. The factors which relate to these instances of repetition may furnish a lead to the means of their curtailment. The fact that "language maturity" does not appear to relate to amounts of repetition simplifies the problem in that one possible assumption of a source of influence on repetitions may be eliminated.

Assuming that situations, as described and as related in this study to repetitions, are important to the fluency of the speech of children of preschool age, the preventive and therapeutic problems become then matters of the manipulation of the environment. Such a view is far from new, but has been reflected for years in the remedial work done by those speech correctionists who favored a psychological approach to the problem of the correction of nonfluent speech. The results of this study give a small amount of weight in favor of such an approach and in addition avoid in slight measure ambiguity and interpretative uncertainty by eliminating generalized emotional descriptions such as "fear," "thwarting," etc. It is often asking the impossible to suggest to a parent that he alter the home environment to give the child more "security" with a minimum of "thwarting" experiences present. It is possible, though, to suggest to parents that they listen, that is, give their attention to the child, when addressed by him with the hope on the part of the clinician that it may be done. It is possible to tell parents to attend when the child wishes to have them do something, being careful that refusals to act in the manner wished are handled in an adult fashion so that the child does not build "tensions" over situations of asking favors of the parents.

The writer is aware of the many limitations of the portion of the study dealing with situations. Too great generalization from the preschool situation to the home might be dangerous. Future research might attempt an uncovering of repetition-fostering situations in other environments with the view to seeing how much overlapping there is from one environment to another. With such information at hand it might be possible to list "danger-points" of child management which have their significance reflected in the degree of fluency of the child's speech.

LANGUAGE PATTERNS OF PRE-SCHOOL CHILDREN
Mary Shattuck Fisher
Sarah Lawrence College and
Columbia University

The purpose of this study is to investigate the following questions:
1. What are the relations between the language patterns of the pre-school child and his age, sex, and intelligence?
2. What do these patterns show about his relative interest in himself, in other persons, and in material objects?
3. What are the social implications of these patterns?

SUBJECTS

The data on which this study is based were obtained from stenographic records of approximately nine hours of language for each of seventy-two pre-school children in the nursery school of the Child Development Institute of Teachers College, Columbia University. The records were taken during the two school years from September, 1928, to June, 1930. There was no basis for selecting the children except that they happened to be enrolled in the nursery school of the Child Development Institute at the time the study was begun. The entire group of seventy-two, composed of thirty-seven girls and thirty-five boys, ranged in age from twenty-two to sixty months. For purposes of analysis the subjects were divided into six month age levels, even though the distribution according to age levels was not constant. Furthermore, the group was highly selected as indicated by a mean IQ of 136.

METHOD OF OBSERVATION

All language records used were taken in the normal nursery school environment. On

JOURNAL OF EXPERIMENTAL EDUCATION, 1932, Vol. 1, pp.70-85.

the three different days when his language
was being recorded, each child was followed
by a trained stenographer from the moment he
arrived in the morning until he finished his
lunch and was ready to enter the sleeping
room for his afternoon nap. All vocalizations or remarks made during this time were
recorded for each child exactly as they
sounded to the stenographer. Records were not
used until a practice period had determined
the efficiency of the stenographer in recording children's language.

The literature in the field of children's
language is rich and extensive. Unfortunately, it is difficult to evaluate the results
because of the wide variation in methodology.
The social implications of language development have, for the most part, been neglected or misinterpreted because of the peculiar
problems connected with gathering and analyzing such material. Large samples of the
spontaneous language of pre-school children
taken under natural yet controlled situations and by a controlled method are extremely difficult to collect. The present
investigation has attempted to satisfy these
requirements which a study of language in
the social field implies.

The following factors helped assure adequacy of the samples in the present study:
(1) the length of time of observation (nine
to twelve hours) for each subject; (2) the
variety of situations in which language was
recorded for each child; and (3) the recording of both spontaneous responses and responses elicited by others in each situation.

The fact that all the children whose language was studied were responding to the
same material and social stimuli in the same
nursery school situations has made comparison of their language patterns possible and
defensible. It would have been more satis-
factory if the number in each age group had
been constant. The importance, however, of
having the records all taken in the same environment outweighed other considerations
for the purpose of this study.

TECHNIQUE OF ANALYSIS
The method of analysis also is different

from that used by previous investigators.
One of the main purposes of the study was to
develop an objective technique for the
analysis of children's language. The following categories for the purpose of
analysis were developed and were found to
satisfy the criteria of objectivity:

1. Grammatical form, independent of
thought content, was used as an indication
of the various stages through which children pass in gaining linguistic control.

2. The sentence, as one unit of vocal expression was used as a logical basis for
consideration and analysis of the language.
The data were recorded so that kinds of
sentences used (simple, compound, complex,
and compound-complex) appeared to indicate
stage and complexity of sentence structure
at different age levels.

3. Sentences were also analyzed to fall
into four categories which indicated the degree of egocentricity and socialization of
the child. The categories are:

    I - Self as subject of sentence
    II - Other person as subject of sentence
    III - Thing as subject of sentence
    IV - Non-verbal or incomprehensible re-
        marks

The method of analysis just described was
developed in order that it might justify an
attempt to see at different age levels:

1. What proportion of the speech of pre-
school children tends to be non-verbal?

2. What proportion tends to be exact
repetition?

3. What proportion tends to be incomplete
as far as sentence structure is concerned?

4. What proportion tends to be about the
self as compared to other persons or
material objects, as indicated by the
subjects of the sentences?

The quantitative measures obtained for
each child were grouped and analyzed under
three heads: construction analysis, functional analysis, and social indices. A brief
discussion and summary of results follows.
For detailed discussion the reader is referred to the published monograph.[1]

1. Language Patterns of Pre-school Children, Child Development Monograph, Teachers College, Columbia University.
(In press).

It is well known that early childhood is the period of most rapid growth in language. At six years of age normal children have acquired all the ordinary speech patterns used by the adults about them, even though their reasoning still remains naive. From the developmental point of view these adult speech patterns emerge out of the incomprehensible babbling of infancy with amazing rapidity. For the children studied, the percentage of non-verbal remarks in total remarks ranged from 45 to one per cent from the beginning of the second year to the beginning of the fifth year. The mean percentage for the entire group was eight per cent. The amount of non-verbal speech was negatively correlated with age. (Pearson r equals $-.42 \pm .07$.)

The sex difference was marked. At all age levels, the boys studied used a higher percentage of incomprehensible remarks than the girls did. Part of this difference is accounted for by a greater tendency on the part of boys to indulge in dramatic play which calls for shouts, hoots, and jungle sounds in general. In spite of the small number of cases, the difference found between the sexes in this respect has some degree of statistical reliability, there being 90 chances in 100 of a true difference. (Ratio of the difference to the probable error of the difference is 1.95.)

The percentage of exact repetition in total remarks gave further interesting sex and age patterns. Repetition was defined as exact repetition of the same remark, verbal or non-verbal, with no variation in word or sound pattern. The correlation between chronological age and per cent of exact repetition in total remarks was significant $(-.73 \pm .04)$. Thus the tendency to repeat the same sound over and over was found to decrease with age. There were, however, marked individual differences. One interesting side light on this habit of repetition was suggested by the fact that a large proportion of the exact repetitions was found to have occurred in the questions being asked adults. Faced with an unheeding

adult the young child seems to be under a
repetitive compulsion. The boys studied repeated themselves more than the girls, with
74 chances in 100 of there being a true difference.

The next developmental pattern to be
considered was that of sentence structure.
For purposes of this analysis the incomplete
sentence category included all structurally
incomplete remarks, regardless of whether or
not the sentences were functionally complete.
This was done in the interest of objectivity. There was found to be a significant
negative correlation between chronological
age and the per cent of incomplete sentences
in total remarks. (Pearson r equals -.73 $\pm$
.03.) No significant correlation was found
between percentage of incomplete remarks and
IQ. At all age levels the girls studied used
a greater proportion of structurally complete sentences in their total speech.

When these structurally complete sentences
were analyzed by themselves, very definite
developmental patterns were indicated. All
children studied were using some complete
sentences. For the entire group the percentage of complete sentences in total speech
ranged from 10 to 89 per cent. For the children under two years of age, all complete
sentences used were simple sentences. The
first instance of a compound sentence in
these records occurred at twenty-four months.
After thirty-four months no child studied
failed to use compound sentences. The first
complex sentence was used at twenty-seven
months. After thirty-two months no child
failed to use some complex sentences. The
first compound-complex sentence in these records occurred at twenty-nine months, and after forty-nine months all subjects were
using such sentences. Thus by the beginning
of the fourth year, the children of this
highly selected group had acquired all ordinary sentence patterns of adults. The use
of complex and elaborated sentences was highly correlated with both chronological age
and IQ, the Pearson r's being .79 $\pm$ .03 and
.84 $\pm$ .02 respectively. The girls, again,
showed consistently superior language development at all age levels. To summarize
structural patterns, the results of this
study suggest that, on the whole, with nor-

mal or superior children age is more important than intelligence in determining the
stage of sentence structure in language development in the pre-school years.

FUNCTIONAL ANALYSIS

The results of the functional analysis
are considered next. Language may be
primarily social in function, but any attempt to limit its purpose to communication
distorts the developmental picture and blots
out discriminating differences in individual
patterns. From the point of view of child
psychology perhaps the most important speech
patterns are those which differentiate individual children with respect to their interests and desires.

The purpose of analyzing the present language records into the functional categories
used has been to gain just such an index.
The relative amount of time that children
spend talking about themselves, compared to
the amount of time they spend talking about
other people or things, was roughly obtained
by dividing sentences into three main categories depending upon the subject of the
sentence. Such a division is obviously arbitrary, and doubtless often violates the
intention or interest of the child. The jus-
tification for using the subject of the
sentence as the criterion for the functional
analysis lies in its objectivity and the
desire to see what patterns, if any, would
be indicated. Very definite and interesting
relationships were indicated in these records when the percentages of remarks in each
category were correlated with chronological
age. There was no relationship whatsoever
between increase in age and amount of talking about self as shown by a Pearson r of
.0002 $\pm$ .08. Instead, the proportion remained constant. It seems safe to infer
that a high degree of concern with himself,
as indicated by the proportion of remarks
made about self, is characteristic of the
pre-school child.

On the other hand, the relationship between increased age and percentage of remarks in Category II (other person as subject) suggested a very different developmental pattern. A high positive relationship

65

was indicated by a Pearson r of .69 ± .04.
The table of means showed a steady and definite increase through the forty-seventh
month and then a slight falling off.

A negative correlation of -.67 ± .04 existed between chronological age and percentage of remarks in Category III (thing as
subject). These data seem to justify the
following conclusions about the child's interests as indicated by the subjects of his
remarks:
(1) After the second year, increase in age
does not bring about an increase in the a-
mount of time a child talks about himself.
The proportion remains constant. (2) The proportion of total remarks about other people
increases with age up to the fourth year.
(3) The proportion of remarks about objects
decreases as age advances up to the fourth
year.

The sex differences were definitely marked.
The boys studied talked more about objects
than did the girls, with 91 chances in 100
of there being a true difference. (The ratio of the difference to the probable error
of the difference is 2.) The girls talked
more about other people than did the boys,
although the reliability of the difference is
not as great. (The ratio of the difference
to the probable error of the difference is
.95.) No sex difference was indicated in
respect to talking about self. The correlations between the percentages in these three
categories (self as subject, other person as
subject, and thing as subject) and IQ were
not reliable enough to be significant.

SOCIAL ANALYSIS

In order to get some measure of true egocentricity and socialization of the child a
coefficient of egocentricity was obtained for
each subject. The proportion of egocentric
remarks to total speech was obtained by dividing total remarks in Category I (self as
subject) by the sum of total remarks in Categories II and III (other person as subject;
thing as subject). The mean coefficient for
the entire experimental group was .53. This
coefficient remained remarkably constant.
That there was no relationship with increase
in age in the pre-school years is indicated

by a Pearson r of .0045. In other words, the
pre-school children studied made a consistently high proportion of their total remarks
about themselves at all age levels. They
talked constantly about what they were doing
from moment to moment.

The amount of speech was also considered a
social index, and showed very definite developmental patterns. For the children studied the average number of remarks was ninety-
two per hour. Marked individual differences
were indicated by a range of 172 remarks per

hour. There was no reliable sex difference.
Amount of speech was positively correlated
with age with a definite and steady increase
up to the forty-eighth month. Then the a-
mount remained fairly constant ($.56 \pm .05$).
The correlation between IQ and amount of
speech was not significant ($.20 \pm .07$).

The percentages of questions and commands
in total speech also gave important developmental patterns as well as social and functional indices. For both questions and commands there was a steady increase in amount
as age advanced, with a definite peak at a-
bout thirty-eight months. After that there
was a slight falling off and a general leveling.

The proportion of negative sentences in
total sentences increased as the children
grew older. The correlation between chronological age and per cent of negative sentences
was $.71 \pm .04$. Negation, as expressed in
language, was greatest during the fourth and
fifth years. No reliable relationship was
found between intelligence and the amount of
verbal negation. As soon as the word no was
learned, it was found to have been used
steadily and fluently throughout all the pre-
school years. There was no significant increase in amount with advance in age, and no
reliable sex difference. Individual differences, however, were marked.

The use of the first personal pronoun in
the plural as an index of social development showed significant age differences ($.72
\pm .04$). There was no significant relation-
ship, however, between IQ and the use of we,
our, and us ($.18 \pm .07$). The girls showed
more rapid social development in this respect than did the boys insofar as use of we,

our, and us suggests increasing awareness of
membership in a large group.

The amount of calling or mentioning children or adults by name was also analyzed.
The amounts did not differ at different ages
nor between the sexes. From the point of
view of children's interests, however, it was
significant that these nursery school children as a group talked to or about children
more than twice as much as they talked to or
about adults.

CONCLUSIONS

Although this investigation made no pre-
tense of being a normative study, based on
a random sampling of the pre-school population, it nevertheless has revealed certain
patterns which are in all probability developmental since all of the indices discussed are more highly correlated with chronological age than with intelligence. It has
seemed evident that among normal and superi-
or children, chronological age is more important than mental age in determining the
various stages of language development.
Girls tend to develop more rapidly than boys.
By the beginning of the fifth year both boys
and girls have acquired all the language patterns commonly used by adults in ordinary
conversation.

The maturity implied in this control of
language and sentence structure is nevertheless misleading. Throughout all the pre-
school years even these superior children
naively continued to experiment with repetitions of sound or word patterns. Even after
control of adult speech forms was acquired
non-verbal or incomprehensible remarks appeared continuously and irrelevantly.

The functional patterns inherent in the
structure of the language indicated much
that is of value about a child's interests
and desires. Revealed through these language patterns, the pre-school child is a
confirmed egotist and yet extremely sociable.
He satisfies both needs by talking incessant-
ly to other people, but telling them of whatever he happens to be doing at the moment.
Gradually, as he grows older, he talks more
and more about other people, but not at the
price of leaving himself out of the picture.

68

Instead, he talks the same amount about himself but less about material objects.   His
interest in other people closely parallels
an increase in the number of commands issued
and the number of questions asked. Perhaps
the most outstanding feature of the language
of the pre-school child as revealed in this
study is the amazing constancy of the coefficient of egocentricity.

   [The "Journal of Experimental Education,"
Volume I, No. 2.]

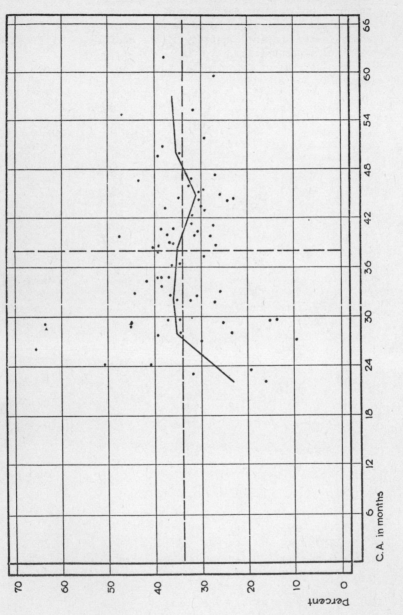

Figure 1

Chronological Age and Per Cent of Remarks in Category I
(Self as Subject)

70

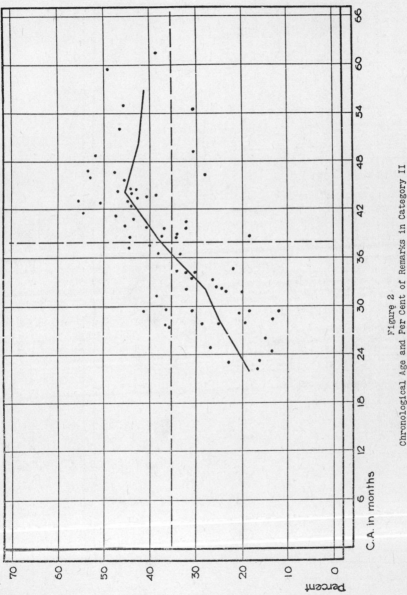

Figure 2
Chronological Age and Per Cent of Remarks in Category II
(Other Person as Subject)

71

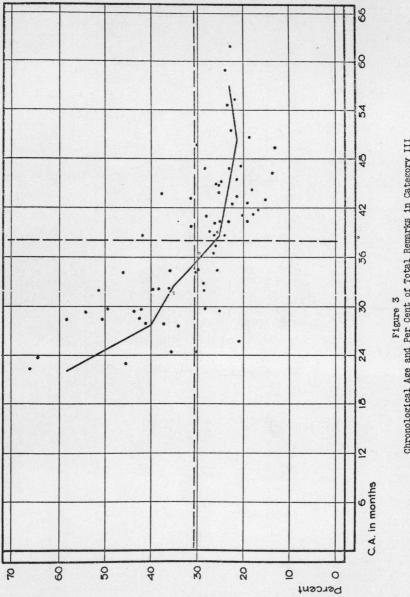

Figure 3

Chronological Age and Per Cent of Total Remarks in Category III
(Thing as Subject)

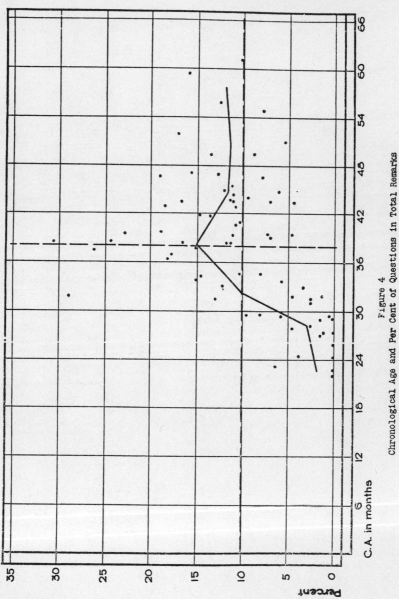

C.A. in months

Figure 4

Chronological Age and Per Cent of Questions in Total Remarks

73

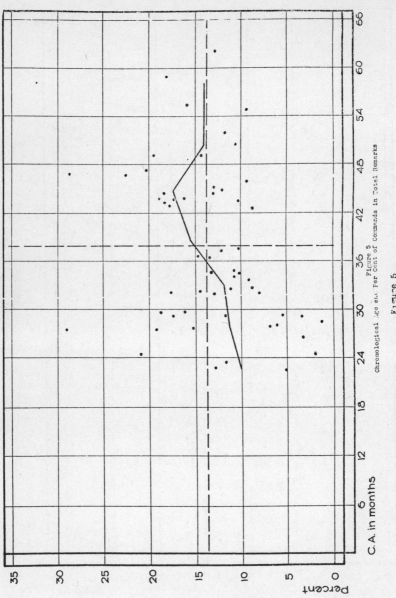

Figure 5

Chronological Age and Per Cent of Commands in Total Remarks

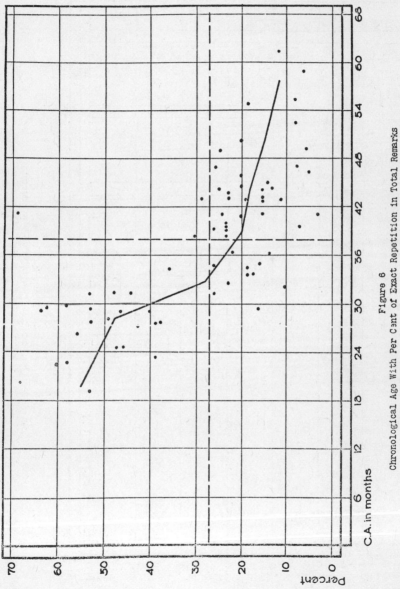

Figure 6

Chronological Age With Per Cent of Exact Repetition in Total Remarks

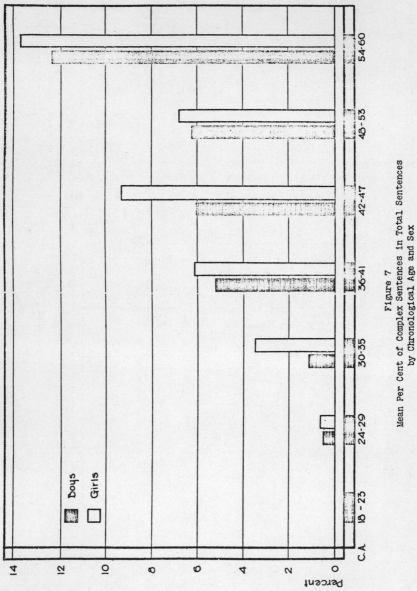

Figure 7

Mean Per Cent of Complex Sentences in Total Sentences
by Chronological Age and Sex

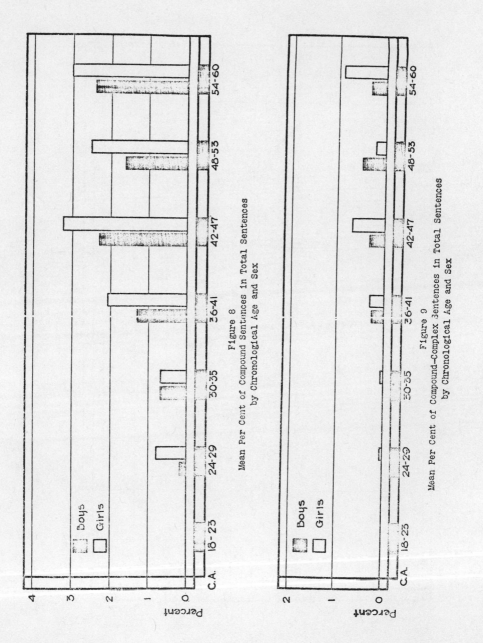

Figure 8

Mean Per Cent of Compound Sentences in Total Sentences
by Chronological Age and Sex

Figure 9

Mean Per Cent of Compound-Complex Sentences in Total Sentences
by Chronological Age and Sex

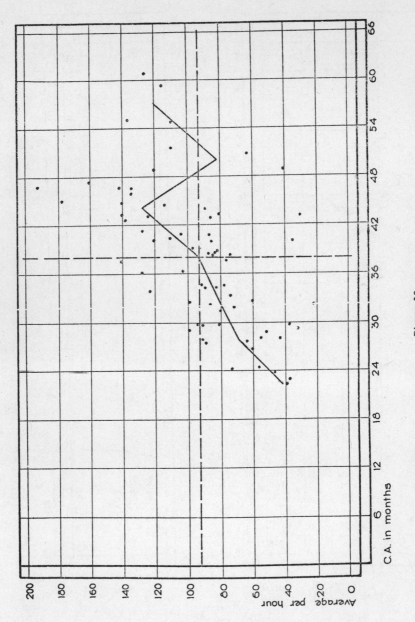

C.A. in months

Average per hour

Figure 10

Chronological Age and Average Remarks Per Hour

78

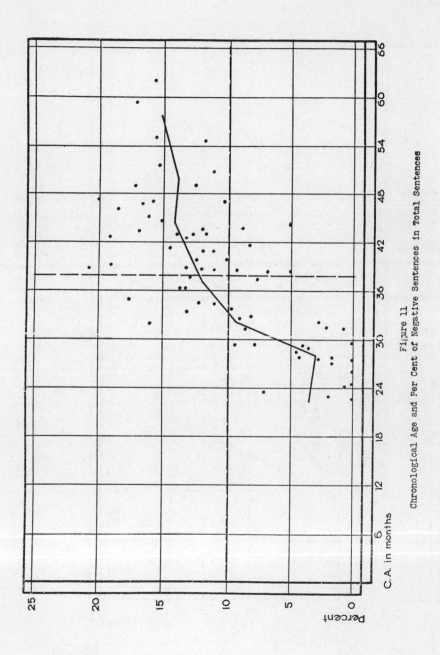

Figure 11

Chronological Age and Per Cent of Negative Sentences in Total Sentences

79

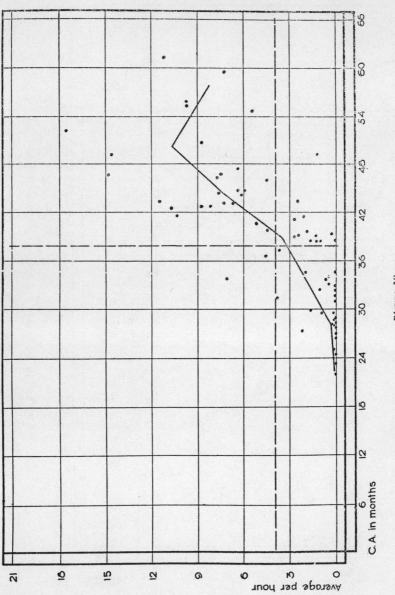

C.A. in months

Average per hour

Figure 12:
Chronological Age and Average Use of Wa, Our, Ua Per Hour

80

Children's Reactions To Nonfluencies In Adult Speech

Thomas G. Giolas

Dean E. Williams

It has been well established that nonfluencies occur in the speech of young children (*3, 5*). Furthermore, Johnson (*4*) has observed that in certain instances these nonfluencies are reacted to or labeled by adults as 'stuttering.' He has hypothesized that stuttering, as a clinical problem, develops after the diagnosis.

Tuthill (7), Bloodstein (*1*) and Boehmler (2) have reported investigations in which they studied the reactions of adults to different types and frequencies of speech nonfluencies. To date no attempt appears to have been made to determine to what extent a child is aware of or reacts to nonfluent speech.

It is recognized that children exhibit a tendency to classify or label one another, as pointed out by Murphy (*6*). If children learn early to classify and label people, events, or actions which they consider 'different,' then it would seem that they might react similarly to certain types of speech nonfluencies. This appears reasonable in view of the fact that they live in a society which often considers certain types of nonfluencies, particularly syllable repetition, as being 'different' or 'abnormal.'

An important consideration, therefore, is to determine whether children react to nonfluencies in the speech of others and, if so, whether their reactions are favorable or unfavorable. If it can be demonstrated that they react unfavorably, it might be assumed that they not only may react to, and label as 'different,' the nonfluencies which occur in the speech of others but that they may also react similarly to those which occur in their own speech.

It was the purpose of this study to determine whether specific kinds of nonfluencies influence a child's preference for (1) a particular story or (2) a particular person telling a story. In addition, an evaluation was made of the extent to which the children referred to the speech nonfluencies in giving reasons for their preferences.

Procedure

Thomas G. Giolas (M.A., Indiana University, 1956) is Graduate Research Assistant in Audiology and Speech, University of Pittsburgh. Dean E. Williams (Ph.D., State University of Iowa, 1952) is Assistant Professor of Speech and Theatre, Speech and Hearing Clinic, Indiana University.

Subjects. The subjects were 120 kindergarten and second-grade children, ranging in age from five years and five months to eight years. They were divided approximately equally as

JOURNAL OF SPEECH AND HEARING RESEARCH, 1958, Vol. 1 , pp. 86-93.

to sex. No child was included who had a speech defect or a history of speech therapy or who had had in his classroom a person diagnosed as a 'stutterer.'

Reading Passages. Three 250-word reading passages were composed. These stories were evaluated by personnel of the Indiana University Reading Clinic as being comparable in subject matter, suitable in content in terms of grade level and equal in comprehension difficulty. Parity of interest level was determined by reading the three stories to 19 second-grade children. Of these children, seven selected Story 1 as their favorite, six preferred Story 2 and six chose Story 3, indicating that there was no tendency to select a particular story in preference to any other.

Types of Nonfluencies. Three copies of each of the stories were prepared. One contained no modifications and was identified as the Fluent Pattern. A second copy was modified so that a predetermined number and kind of interjections were embodied in the passage. This was called the Interjections Pattern. The number of interjections inserted corresponded to 10 per cent of the total number of words in each story. The following three kinds of interjections were inserted randomly through each passage: [ə], [ɑ], and [ʌ]. A table of random numbers was used to determine the dispersion of interjections throughout each passage. The third copy, identified as the Repetitions Pattern, was modified to include a predetermined number of repetitions of the initial portion of certain words. Half of the nonfluencies were two-syllable and half were three-syllable repetitions,

for example, 'b- b- boy' and 'b- b- b-boy.' Again interruptions were 10 per cent of the total number of words in each story, and they were located randomly as in the Interjections Pattern.

The Fluent Pattern was used as a control; the Interjections Pattern represented a type of nonfluency which might or might not be evaluated as 'stuttering'; and the Repetitions Pattern represented a type which is often diagnosed as 'stuttering' (2).

Method of Recording. Three female speech clinicians were rehearsed in their reading of the stories until each speaker could produce the stories using each of three patterns. The Fluent Pattern was rehearsed until it could be read without any observable breaks in the rhythm of speech. Both the Interjections Pattern and the Repetitions Pattern were practiced until the correct number and kind of nonfluencies could be inserted into the passage without noticeable change in the reading rate or inflection pattern. Three trained speech correctionists judged each reading as adequate. Tape-recordings were then made of the stories with the speakers, the stories and the patterns rotated to provide for a recording of each story with each of the patterns by at least two speakers.

The Experiment. The experiment consisted of two parts. Part I was designed to study the effect of a specific fluency pattern upon story preference. Thirty-six second-grade children were divided into three experimental groups. No two groups heard the stories in the same order, nor was the same story presented to any two groups with the same fluency pattern.

TABLE 1. Distribution of frequencies of choices by 36 second-grade children of story content and results of the chi-square test.

Stories	Choices			Chi-square*
	1st	2nd	3rd	
1	8	16	12	2.67
2	14	8	14	2.00
3	14	11	10	.75

*A chi-square value of 5.99 ($df = 2$) is required for significance at the five per cent level.

The recordings were played in a quiet room to the children in groups of six. They were told that they would hear three stories and that they were to listen closely as they would be asked to name the story they liked best. The title of each story was announced and the three recordings were then played. The following questions were then asked each child privately:

1. Which story did you like the best?
2. Which story did you like next best?
3. (a) Then you put this story (the remaining story was named) last. Why did you put it last?
   (b) Why didn't you like the last story?
   (c) Didn't you like the story or didn't you like the way it was told? Why?

The children's responses to each question were recorded verbatim. The three parts of Question 3 were structured in such a way that they became progressively more specific and that the suggestion introduced to a degree in part (b) and to a greater degree in part (c) would not affect the answers to the preceding parts.

Part II was designed to study the effect of a particular fluency pattern upon a child's preference for a specific speaker. Subjects were 36 additional second-grade children and 30 kindergarten children. The children listened to the same story three times, presented each time by a different speaker using a different fluency pattern. The recordings were played in a quiet room to the children in groups of six. The order of presentation for the three speakers was uniformly rotated from group to group. In each instance the children were instructed that they would hear three ladies telling the same story and that they were to decide which lady they would like for a teacher. Each child was then asked the following questions in private:

1. Which lady would you like to have for a teacher? Why did you pick that lady?
2. If you could have two teachers, which lady would you pick second (or next)? Why?
3. Now, you didn't pick the lady—(the third choice was mentioned). Can you tell me why you didn't pick her?

The responses were recorded verbatim.

Results

Part I. The chi-square test, under the hypothesis of chance distribution

TABLE 2. Distribution of frequencies of choices by 36 second-grade children of speech patterns and results of the chi-square test.

Patterns	Choices			Chi-square*
	1st	2nd	3rd	
Fluent	12	8	16	2.67
Interjections	9	15	12	1.50
Repetitions	15	13	8	2.17

*A chi-square value of 5.99 ($df = 2$) is required for significance at the five per cent level.

of choices, was used to evaluate the effect upon the story preferences of the following variables: (1) the story content, (2) the speech pattern used in telling the story, and (3) the position (first, second or third) in which the stories were presented.

Table 1 presents the distribution of first, second and third choices of each story content. Chi-square test results provided no evidence of differences among first, second and third choices for any story content.

Table 2 shows the distribution of first, second and third choices of each of the patterns, identified as Fluent, Interjections and Repetitions Patterns. Chi-square results were not significant and provided no evidence that any one of the patterns affects the distribution of first, second and third choices of stories.

TABLE 3. Distribution of frequencies of choices by 36 second-grade children of positions of story presentation and results of the chi-square test.

| Positions | Choices | | | Chi-square* |
	1st	2nd	3rd	
1	4	9	23	16.17
2	19	10	7	6.50
3	13	17	6	6.00

*Chi-square values of 5.99 and 9.21 ($df = 2$) are required for significance at the five and the one per cent levels, respectively.

The distribution of first, second and third choices for each of the three positions of story presentation is shown in Table 3. Chi-square results were significant in each instance. An examination of the distributions shows that first position was least favored. Each story, however, was heard an equal number of times in each position and the different patterns were used in each position. The only apparent explanation is that the story presented first had either been largely forgotten or had lost much of its interest.

The question of whether the position variable may have obscured other differences, particularly with respect to speech fluency patterns, cannot be answered from these data.

The responses, however, to the questions about the least preferred story indicated that many children were aware of the speech patterns and referred to them as the reason for selection or non-selection of a specific story. The responses were analyzed to determine how many made a reference to the story, the speaker or the manner in which the story was told when stating reasons for designating a given story as *third* choice. All answers were considered compositely, regardless of which speech pattern was employed in relating the story.

To Question 3(a), 'Why did you put it last?' 12 of the 36 children answered, 'I don't know,' and 17 made some reference to the story. Seven referred to the story teller and the way the story was told. Of these seven, three made direct reference to the speech pattern, stating that 'She talked funny,' 'They said um, um, um' and 'One went uh, uh, uh, and she stuttered.'

In response to Question 3(b), 'Why didn't you like the last story?' only two subjects gave no reasons for their preferences. Seventeen referred to the story and 17 made reference to the speech pattern or narrator. The latter made such remarks as 'Because she said uh, uh, uh,' 'She talked funny and silly' and 'She stuttered.'

Question 3(c), 'Didn't you like the story, or didn't you like the way it was told?' suggested to the child a choice of two reasons for his selection, the second of which implied a speaker preference. Three children were undecided or gave ambiguous answers and 11 gave answers which referred to the story. Twenty-two children specified the story teller or speech pattern with such references as 'She talked an, an, an, like that,' 'She stuttered,' 'She pronounced all the words funny' and 'I like the story but she talked funny.'

The children's answers were also analyzed with reference to each of the fluency patterns. Five of the 16 children selecting the story told with the Fluent Pattern as their third choice made no mention of the speech pattern in their replies. The remaining 11 did refer to the speech pattern as the reason for their choice in response to at least one of the three questions. Surprisingly, four of these stated that the speaker 'stuttered.'

The story told with the Interjections Pattern was third choice for 12 children. Four made no reference to the speech pattern and eight mentioned it.

All but one of eight children who rated the story with the Repetitions Pattern third made direct reference to the speech pattern. Two mentioned 'stuttering' specifically.

At times it was observed that a child appeared unsure of the story to which he was referring, sometimes making comments about a story which did not correspond to the speech pattern used in telling that story. Regardless of the questionable reliability of their memories, the reasons given by the children for their selections do indicate that some of them reacted to the speech interruptions.

Part II. The chi-square test, under the hypothesis of chance distribution

TABLE 4. Distribution of frequencies of choices by 36 second-grade children of speakers and results of the chi-square test. Each of three speakers used a different speech pattern.

| Patterns | Choices | | | Chi-square* |
	1st	2nd	3rd	
Fluent	31	4	1	45.50
Interjections	3	24	9	19.50
Repetitions	2	8	26	26.00

*A chi-square value of 9.21 ($df = 2$) is required for significance at the one per cent level

of choices, was used to evaluate the effect of three speech patterns (Fluent, Interjections and Repetitions Patterns) on the preferences of children for a speaker. As indicated previously the children listened to the same story presented by three speakers, each using a different pattern and with position of speakers (or patterns) counterbalanced.

Table 4 presents the distribution of choices by 36 second-grade children for each speaker (or pattern). Significant results of the chi-square tests and the distributions of choices provide evidence that second-grade children will rank the Fluent Pattern as first choice, the Interjections Pattern as second choice and the Repetitions Pattern as third choice.

TABLE 5. Distribution of frequencies of choices by 30 kindergarten children of speakers and results of the chi-square test. Each of three speakers used a different speech pattern.

| Patterns | Choices | | | Chi-square* |
	1st	2nd	3rd	
Fluent	21	5	4	18.20
Interjections	3	12	15	7.80
Repetitions	6	13	11	2.60

*Chi-square values of 5.99 and 9.21 ($df = 2$) are required for significance at the five and the one per cent levels, respectively.

Distributions of choices by 30 kindergarten children, along with results of the chi-square tests, are given in Table 5. Apparently kindergarten children also strongly favor the Fluent Pattern. Differences among frequencies of first, second and third choices are significant for the Interjections Pattern, but not for the Repetitions Pattern. An examination of the distributions, however, provides no evidence that kindergartners prefer one of these patterns to the other.

Twenty-eight of the 36 second-graders made at least one direct reference to a fluency pattern in answering the questions. Fourteen of the 31 children who preferred the speaker using the Fluent Pattern made direct reference to the speech pattern. Typical comments were 'She didn't stutter,' 'She didn't say words over and over again' and 'She didn't say uh, uh, uh.' Qualitative statements included comments that she 'talked,' 'sounded' or 'told' the story 'nice,' 'best,' 'right' or 'good.'

Eight of the 24 second-graders who placed the speaker using the Interjections Pattern second referred directly to the speech pattern. Common comments were of a descriptive nature, such as, 'She just said uh, uh, uh.' Fourteen children commented on the way in which the story was told, with responses such as, 'She wasn't so bad,' 'She just forgot what to say' and 'She just couldn't think it up but she got it out.' Many of the children seemed to classify this pattern as less desirable than the Fluency Pattern and more desirable than the Repetitions Pattern, with comments such as, 'I'd rather have her say uh, uh, uh than stutter,' 'She wasn't so bad,' 'Well, the third one (Repetitions Pattern) was real bad,' or 'The second one (Interjections Pattern) was almost like the first (Fluent Pattern).'

Four of the 26 second-graders who placed the Repetitions Pattern third gave ambiguous reasons or no reasons. The remaining 22 gave the following kinds of reasons: nine classified the pattern as 'stuttering'; 11 described the pattern by referring to the repetitions; and two evaluated the narrator's way of telling the story.

The comments made by the kindergarten children were less specific than those of the second-graders. They more frequently made qualitative statements about the speaker, the speaker's voice or the way the story was told. Only 12 of the 30 children referred directly to the speech pattern in answering the questions. Twenty-one preferred the speaker employing the Fluent Pattern. Of these, only two made direct reference to the patterns, one saying, 'The others said uh, uh, uh, and wa, wa' and the other saying, 'The others kept saying things over and over.' Fourteen made qualitative statements about the speaker. These were similar to those made by the second-graders.

The story teller simulating the Interjections Pattern was the second choice of 12 kindergarten children and the third choice of 15. The speaker employing the Repetitions Pattern was placed second by 13 and third by 11 kindergartners. Only five children specifically mentioned the speech pattern in answering the questions. For the most part the others offered value judgments, such as, 'I didn't like her' and 'She wasn't as good.' The reasons also included descriptive statements such as, 'She talked funny' and 'She sounded like Porky Pig.'

The possibility that preferences might have been influenced by individual differences among speakers other than the simulated speech patterns was considered. An additional group of 18 second-grade children listened to the story with each speaker using a different pattern from the one used previously. All 18 children selected the speaker with the Fluent Pattern as first choice. It was concluded, therefore, that differences among speakers unrelated to the simulated patterns were unimportant in the choices, particularly with respect to the Fluency Pattern.

Discussion

No evidence was obtained that the speech patterns employed in relating the stories affect children's preferences for stories. However, when children are asked to select a person as a prospective teacher, the speech pattern employed does appear to be a determining factor in the selections. The negative finding with respect to the effect of speech pattern upon story selection should thus be interpreted with caution. If speech patterns affect choice of teacher, it seems reasonable to assume that they also affect choice of story. It seems quite possible that the negative finding is the result of the order in which the stories were told, since position did significantly affect the choices.

The second-grade children rated the relative desirability of the three speech patterns with higher agreement than did the kindergartners. They placed the Fluent Pattern first, the Interjections Pattern next and the Repetitions Pattern last. The second-graders were more specific also in giving reasons for their preferences. They more often employed the label 'stuttering.' They were more specific in stating a dislike for speech interruptions, particularly those consisting of repetitions. Most of the kindergartners, however, considered the nonfluent patterns less desirable than

the fluent pattern, but they were less consistent in choosing between the two nonfluent patterns. Their comments, however, indicated that many of them were aware of the speech interruptions and that generally they did not approve of them, although they were somewhat vague in stating their reasons for this disapproval. Apparently, reactions against nonfluencies in the speech of adults were quite general at both age levels.

This study was primarily concerned with children's reactions to and evaluations of the speech of adults. It is possible that the speech standards a child maintains for adults differ from those he maintains for himself or his peers. It seems likely, however, on the basis of the results of this study that children reflect, at a relatively early age, society's critical attitude toward nonfluencies in speech, particularly with reference to repetitions. Inasmuch as children appear to be aware of and to react to the nonfluencies in the speech of others, it seems possible that certain children may, on the basis of socially learned value judgments, react adversely to similar types of nonfluencies in their own speech. This apparent reaction in young children should be given due consideration in any clinical or experimental study of the conditions affecting a child's early reactions to nonfluencies in his own speech.

Summary

The purpose of this study was to determine whether specific kinds of nonfluencies, repetitions and interjections, in the speech of adults influence children's preferences for (1) a story and (2) a person telling a story. The subjects, or listeners, were kindergarten and second-grade children. The experimental material consisted of three stories told by three adult narrators with three speech patterns identified as Fluent, Interjections and Repetitions, respectively.

The results provided evidence that speech patterns affect children's preferences for a person telling a story, but no evidence that they affect preferences for a story.

The children's answers to a questionnaire indicated that they were, in general, aware of the nonfluencies and that they reacted against them.

References

1. BLOODSTEIN, O., JAEGER, W. and TUREEN, J., A study of the diagnosis of stuttering by parents of stutterers and nonstutterers. *JSHD*, 17, 1952, 308-315.

2. BOEHMLER, R. M., A quantitative study of the extensional definition of stuttering with special reference to the audible designata. Ph.D. Dissertation, State University of Iowa, 1953.

3. DAVIS, D. M., The relation of repetitions in the speech of young children to certain measures of language maturity and situational factors; part 1. *JSHD*, 4, 1939, 303-318.

4. JOHNSON, W., A study of the onset and development of stuttering. *JSHD*, 7, 1942, 251-257.

5. JOHNSON, W., *Stuttering in Children and Adults.* Minneapolis: University of Minnesota Press, 1955.

6. MURPHY, G., *Personality: A Biosocial Approach to Origins and Structure.* New York: Harper and Brothers, 1947.

7. TUTHILL, C. E., A quantitative study of extensional meaning with special reference to stuttering. *Speech Monographs*, 13, 1946, 81-98.

PRIMARY STUTTERING AT THE ONSET OF STUTTERING: A REEXAMINATION OF DATA

JAMES R. McDEARMON

Washington State University, Pullman, Washington

This reexamination of certain data in Study III of Johnson's *The Onset of Stuttering* found that: (1) Among experimentals, children labeled as stutterers by at least one parent, at least 63% at onset time evidenced "primary stuttering" (simple repetitions and prolongations of sounds and syllables), and at least 28% evidenced only "normal nonfluencies" (repetitions of words and phrases, and other interruptions common in children), as indicated by parents' responses to one question. (2) This "primary stuttering" was much more frequent, and "normal nonfluency" much less frequent, in experimentals at onset of stuttering than in controls; and these differences were statistically significant. (3) Slight tension was the only "secondary" reaction indicated in more than 15% of the experimentals at onset, according to parents' responses to other questions. At onset experimentals and controls were significantly differentiated in incidence of tension, but not in incidence of indifference, awareness, or irritation. "Secondary" reactions in experimentals showed considerable increase within an average of about 18 months after apparent onset. This study supports the concept of primary stuttering as a beginning phase of a severity continuum.

Two major kinds of arguments have been directed against the concept of primary stuttering. One is that primary stuttering is not sufficiently distinguishable from normal nonfluency. The other is that it is not sufficiently distinguishable from secondary stuttering. According to the first position, the nonfluencies of primary stuttering are too similar to those of normal speech to permit valid differentiation (Johnson, 1956, p. 61). According to the second position, the kind of reactions supposedly characteristic of secondary stuttering are too often found in primary stuttering to permit valid differentiation (Bloodstein, 1958, pp. 15-34).

One of the most important relevant studies completed by Johnson and associates was designated as Study III in the book *The Onset of Stuttering* (1959). There were 150 experimentals and 150 controls. Each experimental was considered a stutterer by at least one parent. Information was provided through interviews with the 600 parents. Johnson did not specifically compare the extent of possible primary and secondary stuttering in experimentals and controls. He did compare the groups as to specific kinds of nonfluencies, and stressed the fact of the overlapping of the groups in the kinds of nonfluencies they exhibited (p. 133).

JOURNAL OF SPEECH AND HEARING RESEARCH, 1968, Vol. 11, pp. 631-637.

"Normal nonfluency" reaction	Repetition of word, phrase, sentence; pause between words; interjection; inability to express thought.
"Primary stuttering" reaction	Simple repetition or prolongation of sound or syllable without complicating characteristics.
"Secondary stuttering" reaction	Block, inability to finish sentence, pause in middle of word, gasp.
Other reaction	Slurring of word, accented word.

Classifying each single reaction was preliminary to classifying each child's overall reported nonfluency pattern on the following basis:

"Normal nonfluency" pattern	"Normal nonfluency" but no "primary" or "secondary" stuttering reactions.
"Primary stuttering" pattern	Case 1. "Primary stuttering" reactions only. Case 2. Both "primary stuttering" and "normal nonfluency" reactions.
"Secondary stuttering" pattern	Case 1. "Secondary stuttering" reactions only. Case 2. Both "secondary" and other reactions.
Other pattern	No "normal nonfluency," "primary," or "secondary" reactions.

Responses to the 11 other questions above provided the remaining raw data used in the present study. These responses were evaluated for presence or absence of "secondary" reactions. All computations were based upon "definite" responses, as indicated by Johnson's data. Computations for significance of difference utilized the chi-square test with Yates's correction. Sets of responses by fathers and mothers were always treated separately, except in Figure 1 where percentages of fathers' and mothers' responses were averaged. Where a single value is given in the results or discussion below to represent both percentages of responses by fathers and mothers, the figure given is the smaller of the two percentages, unless otherwise indicated.

RESULTS

Analysis of responses to questions 217 and 293 are shown in Tables 1, 2, and 3. Table 1 shows numbers and percentages of controls with patterns of normal

TABLE 1. Numbers and percentages of controls indicated, on the basis of definite answers to question 217 by fathers and mothers respectively, as exhibiting "normal nonfluency," "primary stuttering," or "secondary stuttering" patterns, as defined in present study.

Pattern	Indicated by Fathers		Indicated by Mothers	
	Number	%	Number	%
Normal nonfluency	64	92.75	69	86.25
Primary stuttering	4	5.80	10	12.50
Secondary stuttering	1	1.45	1	1.25
Total in Definite Answers	69		80	
Total Subjects	150		150	

My study reexamined some of Johnson's impressive body of data with particular consideration of four questions:

(1) What was the incidence of "normal nonfluency" and "primary stuttering" indicated in the control group?
(2) What was their indicated incidence in the experimental group?
(3) Were the two groups significantly different in these respects?
(4) To what extent was "secondary stuttering" indicated in the control group and in the experimental group?

METHOD

Data concerning parents' responses to 13 questions in Johnson's Study III of *The Onset of Stuttering* were reexamined. These questions are listed below, preceded by their original numbers and, in parentheses, the pages in the appendix containing the questions and the relevant response data:

217 (64-69): Imitate and describe what the child was doing in his speech when he first stuttered—the very first time you noticed the child stuttering, or during the period when the stuttering still was the same as it had been the very first time it was noticed by anybody.

243 (79): When stuttering was first noticed was it accompanied by any grimaces or bodily contortions?

244 (79): Did he seem indifferent to his very first stoppages?

245 (79-80): When the stuttering was first noticed, did the child seem to be aware of the fact that he was speaking in a different manner or doing something wrong?

246 (80): Did the child show surprise or bewilderment after having had trouble on a word?

247 (80): Did the very first stoppages seem to be unpleasant to the child?

248 (80): Do you think the child felt irritated when the very first stoppages occurred?

250 (80-81): At the time when stuttering was first noticed, was the child using force or more effort than usual "to get his words out"? Was there more than usual muscular tension?

251 (81): What was the child's own *first* reaction to the trouble he was having saying words?

293 (94-98): Describe and imitate the present pattern of stuttering.

296 (99-100): How does he react now when he has a lot of trouble saying a word?

305 (104): When the child stutters does he make any grimaces or odd bodily movements, or does he seem to do anything else out of the ordinary?

318 (109): How sensitive was the child about his speech defect?

At the outset of the present study "primary stuttering" was defined as repetitions and prolongations of sounds and syllables without awareness, struggle, tension, frustration, fear, or avoidance. "Secondary stuttering" was defined as interruptions in the flow of speech accompanied by struggle, tension, fear, and other maladaptive emotional reactions. "Normal nonfluency" was defined as the relatively effortless and uncomplicated interruptions common in childhood speech.

In evaluating responses to two open-ended questions, 217 and 293, all reported reactions were classified as below for the present study:

TABLE 2. Numbers and percentages of experimentals at onset time indicated, on the basis of definite answers to question 217 by fathers and mothers respectively, as exhibiting "normal nonfluency," "primary stuttering," or "secondary stuttering" patterns, as defined in present study.

Pattern	Indicated by Fathers		Indicated by Mothers	
	Number	%	Number	%
Normal nonfluency	47	32.87	41	28.08
Primary stuttering	91	63.64	98	67.12
Secondary stuttering	5	3.50	7	4.79
Total in Definite Answers	143		146	
Total Subjects	150		150	

nonfluency, primary stuttering, and secondary stuttering, as indicated by responses of fathers and mothers. Table 2 gives parallel information concerning experimentals at onset time. Table 3 gives parallel information concerning experimentals at interview time which, parents indicated, averaged about 18 months after onset time.

On the basis of responses by fathers, the percentages of patterns of normal nonfluency, primary stuttering, and secondary stuttering among controls were about 93, 6, and 1.5 respectively (Table 1); among experimentals at onset, about 33, 64, and 3.5 (Table 2); and among experimentals at interview time, about 15, 77, and 7.5 (Table 3). Percentages based on responses by mothers showed similar trends.

These data are summarized in Figure 1. It shows, on the basis of the means of the percentages indicated by responses of fathers and mothers to questions 217 and 293, the averaged percentages of controls, experimentals at onset, and experimentals at interview time, exhibiting normal nonfluency, primary stuttering, and secondary stuttering patterns.

Values were computed for significance of differences between controls and experimentals at both onset and interview times in (1) incidence of normal nonfluency patterns, and (2) incidence of primary stuttering patterns. All chisquare values for both fathers' and mothers' responses were far beyond that required for significance at the 0.001 level.

TABLE 3. Numbers and percentages of experimentals at interview time indicated, on basis of definite answers to question 293 by fathers and mothers respectively, as exhibiting "normal nonfluency," "primary stuttering," "secondary stuttering," or "other" patterns, as defined in present study.

Pattern	Indicated by Fathers		Indicated by Mothers	
	Number	%	Number	%
Normal nonfluency	22	15.07	23	15.75
Primary stuttering	112	76.71	112	76.71
Secondary stuttering	11	7.53	11	7.53
Other	1	.68	0	
Total in Definite Answers	146		146	
Total Subjects	150		150	

Responses to question 251, concerned with the child's first reaction to trouble saying words, indicated no secondary reactions in at least 86% of the experimentals. In these subjects behavior was described as "no reaction," "laughed," or "kept on trying."

Questions 243 to 248, inclusive, were concerned with specific secondary reactions at onset. The percentages of responses indicating no such secondary reactions among experimentals ranged from about 85 to 95. No significant differences were found between controls and experimentals at onset in reported incidence of indifference, awareness, or irritation. Data did not permit computation by the chi-square method of significance of difference regarding the other reactions.

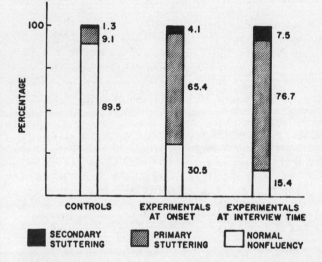

FIGURE 1. Mean percentages of controls and experimentals exhibiting the three types of nonfluency patterns, computed by averaging percentages of responses of fathers and mothers to questions 217 and 293.

However, responses to question 250 indicated a significantly higher incidence of tension and effort in experimentals at onset than in controls at the 0.01 and 0.02 levels. No tension was reported in 64% of the experimentals; no tension more than slight in 85%.

Three questions were particularly concerned with secondary reactions at interview time. Responses to question 318 indicated "not sensitive" with significantly more frequency in controls than in experimentals at the 0.001 level. No sensitivity was reported in 68% of the experimentals; no sensitivity greater than mild in about 86%.

Two open-ended questions, 296 and 305, while indicating that the majority of experimentals were still without secondary reactions at interview time, also indicated an increase in such reactions since onset. The former concerned the child's reactions when having difficulty speaking. No secondary reactions were indicated in at least 60%, whose behavior was reported as "no reaction," "keeps trying," and "laughs." Secondary reactions were indicated in at least 20% by both fathers and mothers.

Question 305 was concerned with grimaces or other unusual movements. No such reactions were indicated in 60%. Secondary reactions were indicated by fathers in 36%, by mothers in 40%.

DISCUSSION

This study indicates that controls and experimentals at onset were strongly differentiated, not only in the incidence of specific nonfluency reactions that Johnson (1959, p. 135) found, but in the incidence of tension, "normal non-fluency," and "primary stuttering." It tends to confirm Van Riper's (1963, p. 328) description of primary stuttering, which specified repetitions and prolongations of sounds and syllables, not pauses or repetitions of words and phrases.

The results also indicate that secondary reactions were relatively infrequent at stuttering onset, but that they began developing shortly afterward. Only one secondary reaction, tension, appeared to have incidence of greater than 15% among experimentals at onset, and tension in excess of "slight" appeared to have no greater than 15% incidence. At interview time secondary reactions appeared to have increased to an incidence of 36% or more, on the basis of responses to one open-ended question.

Considerable discrepancy appeared, among experimentals, between the relatively small frequencies of secondary stuttering patterns indicated by responses to questions 217 and 293, and the much larger frequencies of secondary reactions indicated by responses to other questions. The difference in emphasis of the questions was no doubt influential. Questions 217 and 293, to the unsophisticated interviewee, at least, were worded with apparent emphasis more on reactions in the stuttering; other questions, with the exception of number 250 on "tension," more on reactions to the stuttering.

The high incidence—at least 35%—of varying degrees of tension among experimentals at onset deserves special note. Bloodstein (1960) stressed the frequency of tension in many of the youngest stutterers. These findings about tension and, to a lesser extent, about other secondary reactions, suggest that the concept of "primary stuttering," like most concepts in behavior, is a relative one.

The results of this study tend to support Bloodstein's (1958, pp. 15-34) findings of overlapping and lack of sharp distinction between primary and secondary stuttering, and his finding that primary stuttering, at least in nearly pure form, is by no means universal among stutterers at onset. However, the present results indicate a high incidence, at onset, of sound and syllable repetitions and prolongations, relatively uncomplicated by the reactions of more advanced stuttering. They do not, therefore, support Bloodstein's rejection of the overall distinction between primary and secondary stuttering.

At the same time, these results, while tending to confirm Johnson's findings of overlapping between primary stuttering and normal nonfluency, do not support his rejection of the general distinction between these two behaviors either. Rather, they are in agreement with Wingate's (1962) conclusion, based on a review of a number of studies (including Johnson's Study III), that there exists a difference in kind between nonfluencies of children identified as stutterers and nonfluencies of children not so identified.

The results indicate clearly consistent trends toward increasing severity in the early development of the disorder. Normal nonfluency patterns were much less frequent in experimentals at onset than in controls, still less frequent in experimentals at interview time. Primary stuttering patterns were much more frequent in experimentals at onset than in controls, still more frequent in experimentals at interview time. Secondary reactions, which were more frequent in experimentals at onset time than in controls, increased considerably in experimentals by interview time.

The central findings were: (1) Among experimentals, children labeled as stutterers by at least one parent, at least 63% at onset of stuttering evidenced primary stuttering (simple repetitions and prolongations of sound and syllables), and at least 28% evidenced only normal nonfluencies (repetitions of words and phrases, and other interruptions common in children), as indicated by parents' responses to one question. (2) This primary stuttering was much more frequent, and normal nonfluency much less frequent, in experimentals at onset of stuttering than in controls; and these differences were statistically significant. (3) Slight tension was the only secondary reaction indicated in more than 15% of the experimentals at onset, according to parents' responses to other questions.

These results give a considerable measure of support to the concept of "primary stuttering," although not as a pattern of behavior with more or less definite boundary lines, and not as something almost universal among stutterers at onset. Primary stuttering is rather indicated as a kind of stuttering found in a considerable proportion of stutterers at onset, and as a beginning phase in a continuum of decreasing primary and increasing secondary characteristics.

ACKNOWLEDGMENT

The author gratefully acknowledges the assistance of Ruth Millburn Clark, Professor of Speech, University of Denver, and Katherine Snow Egan, Associate Professor of Speech Pathology and Audiology, Idaho State University, for their critical reading of the manuscript and their comments and suggestions.

REFERENCES

BLOODSTEIN, O., Stuttering as an anticipatory struggle reaction. In J. Eisenson (Ed.), Stuttering: A Symposium. New York: Harper (1958).

BLOODSTEIN, O., The development of stuttering: I. Changes in nine basic features. J. Speech Hearing Dis., 25, 219-237 (1960).

JOHNSON, W., (Summary) In E. F. Hahn and Elise S. Hahn (Eds.), Stuttering: Significant Theories and Therapies. Stanford: Stanford Univ. Press (1956).

JOHNSON, W., The Onset of Stuttering. Minneapolis: Univ. of Minnesota Press (1959).

VAN RIPER, C., Speech Correction. Englewood Cliffs, N.J.: Prentice-Hall (1963).

WINGATE, M. E., Evaluation and stuttering, Part I: Speech characteristics of young children. J. Speech Hearing Dis., 27, 106-115 (1962).

Speech Profiles Of The
Pre-school Child 18 To 54 Months

Ruth W. Métraux

GESELL, IN HIS study of the development of the infant and child (2), has not always confined his analysis to tabulation of details alone, but has attempted to give a dynamic and integrated picture of the child, a picture which reveals the child as he acts and thinks, as he works and plays, a picture of the child as we see him in his many facets of behavior.

Many detailed and well-documented studies have been made of the speech and speech production of the child but, so far as this writer is able to determine, no one has attempted to give a description of the dynamic speech of the child at each age. What does the speech of an 18-monther sound like as he plays, works, and communicates his needs? How does it differ from the speech of the two-year-old? How does the three-year-old differ from the four-year-old in his speech?

Irwin (3) has carried on a concrete and scientific investigation of the speech production of infants at two-month intervals from birth to 30 months. He indicates the number and types of phonemes which should be produced by the average child at each age level. From his study it is known what sounds are used, how many

should be expected at each age, and the relative production of the sound in comparison to the total production. This is an excellent developmental gauge, though he does not tell whether these sounds were used correctly in intelligible and communicative speech after intelligible speech appears.

Wellman, Case, Mengert and Bradbury (7) studied the speech sounds of young children and have given tentative norms on the development of each sound at yearly intervals. Following this Williams made an analytical study of language achievements in pre-school children (8) and a qualitative analysis of the erroneous speech sound substitutions of pre-school children (9).

Proceeding beyond the phonetic development of speech, other investigators such as Fisher (1), McCarthy (4), and Smith (6) have determined how grammar and syntax develop in the speech of the child, while Piaget (5) has given some insight into the inter-relation of the development of language and thought.

All of these gauges are valuable in measuring the speech development of a child, and they are needed as accurate and objective points of reference. When the tabulation is finished and the scales are completed, however, it is still the conviction of this observer that there is no real feeling for

Ruth W. Métraux (M.A. Michigan, 1941) is a member of the staff of the Centro de Investigaciones Sociales, University of Puerto Rico. This study was completed at Yale University.

JOURNAL OF SPEECH AND HEARING DISORDERS, 1950, Vol. 15, pp. 37-53.

the total speech of the child. It is known that certain sounds are difficult for some children to master, more or less the age limit at which the speech of the child should be specific, the order in which the various parts of speech are acquired and mastered, the number of phonemes he should produce at each age, and the parts of speech he should use, but few persons can listen to the speech of the average normal child and tell at approximately what speech age he is functioning.

It is the object of this study to attempt to synthesize some of the things known about the speech of the child at various ages. Up to now the speech has been taken from the child and measured; now it is proposed to give the speech back to the child and see how he uses it to reveal himself.

PROCEDURE

At the Clinic of Child Development[1] of Yale University, over a two year period, a total of 207 children at seven pre-school ages (18 months, 24, 30, 36, 42, 48, and 54 months) have been studied and observed. All of the children were attendants of the Guidance Nursery, all of average or above average intelligence.

For each child a developmental examination (Gesell) was recorded, and a phonetic transcript (International Phonetic Alphabet) was made of all replies and all speech which the child used during the examination. In addition, extensive records of speech, phonetically recorded, were made during his play and activity periods in the Guidance Nursery. All of the observations are implemented with notes regarding his total activity and behavior in each situation. Interview records and the report of the mother regarding the language and speech of the child in the home were also used.

[1]Now the Child Study Center.

From the phonetic speech transcripts on 116 of these children, detailed analysis was made of their speech production of consonants and vowels, and an analysis of substitutions and omissions. The production of initial, medial and final consonants and vowels was analyzed and the substitutions of consonants and vowels in all positions was tabulated. All of these results thus far have served only to confirm or to enlarge the results already published in regard to the speech production of the pre-school child. Only after the addition of many more cases at each age group might it be possible to be any more definitive than is the available literature. The only statement which can be made in this report is that vowel production in the child's speech appears to be more than 90% correct by 30 months and consonant production seems to be 90% or more correct by 54 months.

Thus, leaving aside for the moment any results which have been already well defined by others, a composite view will be given of the speech of the child at each of the seven pre-school ages already indicated. In the analysis of the data, and in constant observation of the children in the nursery groups, certain characteristics were perceived which could be followed through each age, though at some ages one characteristic was often more outstanding than others. None of the items are presented as 'norms'; they are, rather, illustrative of some of the things which can be expected in the speech of the child at that age. This outline should serve only as a basis for these and other speech characteristics which can be observed as the child progresses toward complete speech specificity. Each child will, of course, have his own individuality in speech, but it is felt that each age offers speech patterned enough to be described. It is the purpose here merely to indicate some of the elements of that pattern.

18 Months
(28 children studied)

1. *Pronunciation.* The 18-monther leaves off the beginning and the end of a phrase, but with the use of a proper vowel and a medial consonant, as well as the proper inflection, he can make himself understood. Thus, 'See you later' becomes [iuleɪ], 'here I come too' is [ɪɑkʌmku], 'up in the sky' [ʌbikaɪ], and 'orange juice' [ʊdʊ]. On one-word responses, he often gets the initial consonant with a vowel, but seldom the final consonant. A child with minimal speech at this age will often use one syllable or one word for many things and with a changing inflection make himself perfectly clear. [æ] or [ʌ] may be used to indicate 'What is that?' 'Can I have that?' 'No, not that,' and other expressions.

The 18-monther is very uncertain and inconsistent in his production of almost any word. It is the vowel which is the most changeable when he uses the same word in any given period. Thus, for 'ball' he says [bɔ] then [bɑ] and then perhaps [bʊ]; or for 'baby' [bɛbi], [beɪbi], [bɪbi]. One can also hear syllables which are not translatable speech as such, but which change in the same manner: [dɑdududɑdu] or [dɪdɪdoʊ] and [dɪdʌdɪdɪdʌ].

2. *Voice.* His voice is subject to much change and inconsistency, as is most of his speech production at this age. The control seems very unstable. His voice tends to become high pitched and strained. It may vary in a few seconds from a well-modulated voice to a high pitch, then to a yell, a squeak or a sigh. There is a tendency to upward inflection on ends of words and phrases, which often becomes a high whine. He experiments a great deal with voice and pitch, and there is a variety of vocal overflow with little or no phonetic value, such as a laugh, sigh or whisper.

3. *Repetitions.* He repeats syllables or words more frequently than not. When asking for milk, he may say, [mʌmʌmʌmʌ]. The repetition is easy, unforced repetition which can be terminated by himself or by the response of others.

4. *Relation of language and activity.* Vocalization is usually combined with activity to emphasize what he is doing, as with 'sit' [sɪ], 'rock' [rɑ], 'up' [ʌp], as he performs the activity, or 'more' [moʊ] as he hands his cup for milk.

He also uses vocalization in protest. 'No,' is vigorous; 'mine' [maɪ] is less frequent.

With the 18-monther, however, it is the action which is important, and the vocalization is often suppressed entirely in favor of the movement. The 18-month nursery group as a rule is a very quiet corner vocally. Some 18-monthers may say nothing at all during a developmental examination, apart from an occasional [hɛ], [æ] or [bɔŋ] for emphasis.

5. *Language relation to others.* The 18-monther refers to an adult, teacher or mother quite often for check. He usually refers to them with activity, by showing something, smiling, or by gesture or looking toward the person. There is sometimes minimal vocalization with the activity, but often it is the gesture or the activity itself which communicates his need.

6. *Tensional outlets in language situations.* In any situation demanding

attention, such as the developmental examination, or in 'reading' a book, there is inclined to be motor overflow, in order of prominence, of the lips, tongue, jaw, eyes, head. It must be noted that in this section, observation of the overflow in the head and face region will take precedence since it is often more related to speech, though other bodily overflow will be noted.

The 18-monther, unless disturbed, smiles constantly during the developmental examination, and there is a good deal of smiling in the nursery. He may regard a situation, using only his eyes and facial expression to indicate the correct response, and there will be no verbalization. He protrudes his tongue, and bites it occasionally. He will nod assent, and release an object with his hands, but the word 'yes' is not yet a part of his vocabulary.

7. *Illustrative excerpts.* a. Common Expressions. 'What's that?' [ʌæ], [hʌdæ], [wʌdæ], [ʌsæ]. 'All gone' [ɔgɔ], [ɔlgɑ], [ɔlgɔn].

b. Developmental Examination. Picture card: 'doggie' [gɑgi], 'shoe' [su], 'house' [haʊs], [haʊ], 'bow-wow' [baʊwaʊ], [bouwou], 'clock' [tɑ], [tɑk.]

c. Nursery. Boy: (h o l d i n g out block) 'block' [bɑk]. Drops block and goes to door and tries it. 'The key there' [dɑkidæ]. Goes back to blocks, piles them. 'Dung!' [dʊŋ] as block falls. 'Want to take another' [ɔnʌtak-ʌnoukʌ]. 'This go get around' [tɪgou-gɛtʌwaʊ]. 'Here I come too' [ia-kʌmkʊ].

2nd boy: 'Duh duh tah' [dudʊtɑ]. Voice rises on last syllable. 'High chair' [haɪtʃeɪ], he points out chair to teacher who enters the room. Another teacher leaves and says 'bye' and he responds 'bye' [baɪ]. Goes to revolving disk of another child. 'Wheel'

[ʌi], 'I turn wheel' [aɪtʌʍi]. 'Theh da da' [ðɛdɑdɑ].

3rd boy: With blocks. 'Me want water' [miwawawʌ]. 'Vun, two,' he counts. 'Beek bye, go corner, got the buggy, going bang' [bikbaɪ goukɔn kʌtʌbʌgi ɔŋ bæŋ]. Goes to table for juice. 'Got juice' [gɑdʒus]. 'Bow wang' [baʊwaŋ]. Teacher brings turtle to table. 'Fishie, fishie. Put back in' [fɪsʌfisi ʌbagɛn].

Girl: At table. 'Cookie' [kʌke]. 'I want that chair' [ʌwaæhɛʌ]. She has brought blocks to table and is explaining something to boy. 'Ung ae uneeaw ae ae' [ʌŋæ nɪ ɔæ æ].

24 Months
(37 children studied)

1. *Pronunciation.* Although phrases are still greatly telescoped, there is usually a beginning consonant whenever indicated, even though it may be a substitution for the correct one, and the final consonant is often present. Medial consonants are slighted. Thus, 'nother one' is [nʌwʌn] and 'I'm all through' [ʌmɔfu].

Beginning difficulty with syntax may also complicate the speech production. He may say 'Those are me's' [ouzʌmis], and then 'those are mines' [ðouzʌmaɪnz], or 'falleds out' [fɔdz-aʊt]. [w] substitutions for [r] are strong, and lisping begins to be heard, especially on [s] and [ʃ]. In a short period of observation, the 24-monther will, as at 18 months, often change the pronunciation of any given word, and although the v o w e l continues to change, there is now some consonantal change. For example, one will hear 'ball' as [bɔbɔbɔbɔ] and in a few seconds [bwabwabwabwa], or 'horsie' [hɔsi] then [hɔti], and 'choo-choo' [tutu] will become [tʃutʃu].

2. *Voice.* Some of the 18-month high whining tone still persists, though

in general the pitch is lower and easier. There is some nasality in the tone, especially when the voice is loud. The voice still has an unstable up and down quality. There is some straining, and squealing is still common.

3. *Repetitions.* The 24-monther is now using 'a' [ʌ] before many responses, as on the picture cards or pictorial vocabulary in the developmental examination, and he may repeat [ʌʌ] before he finds the correct response. On comprehension questions he uses 'I' quite often, and this too may be repeated before he frames the answer. There is occasional syllable repetition such as 'wi-wi-wipe my hands' [waɪwaɪwaɪpmaɪ hænz] or 'nuh-nuh ball' [nʌnʌbɔ]. The most common characteristic of repetition at this age is a kind of compulsive repetition of a word or phrase. There is sometimes a variation in the phrase, but it seems necessary to the child to repeat it. With some children the compulsion continues to six or seven repetitions, with others perhaps only twice. Thus a child will say, 'here goes, here goes, here goes' [ʌgouʌgouzʌgouz], or 'a ball, dis a ball, dis a ball, Mom' [ʌbɔdɪsʌbɔdɪsʌbɔmɑm].

4. *Relation of language and activity.* Now the child can sometimes use speech to precede his action. He often announces his intentions before he acts, as 'I'll get it' [ʌdɛtʌt], or 'here goes' [ʌgouz]. 'No' is occasionally used in an attempt to control the situation verbally, though action is still the mainstay of control. We still note the enjoyment of action suited to words as he goes 'up' and 'down' or as he 'bangs' the clay.

5. *Language relation to others.* The child now often asks the adult directly to do something for him, or for an answer to a question. With some children, however, an increased awareness of others will serve to make him quite shy and he will not ask directly for help even though he needs it. In relation to his compatriots he often finds screaming or hitting more effective than speech.

6. *Tensional outlets in language situations.* Eyes are the strongest holding factor at this age and there is little motor overflow at this period. His activity is related to the task at hand and there is little extraneous movement.

7. *Illustrative excepts.* a. Common Expressions. 'Mine' [maɪ], [maɪn]; 'another' [nʌ], [ʌnʌ]; 'I want' [aɪwʌn], [wʌn].

b. Developmental Examination. Picture card: 'cup' [kʌp]; 'shoes' [tsus], [hu]; 'clock' [tlɑk]. Pictorial vocabulary: 'car' [kɑ]; 'hat' or 'hat on' [hæt], [hɛt], [hætɔn]; 'airplane' [ʌrpɛn]; 'a moon' [ʌmun]; 'a knife' [ʌnaɪf]. Test objects: 'nickel' [nɪkʌl]; 'keys' [gis]; 'pencil' [pɛntʌl], [pɛntsɪ], [pɛʔʌl].

c. Nursery. 1st boy: Playing with car. 'Red car' [rɛdkɑ].

2nd boy: Looking at book. 'Dat's a squirrel.' [dætsʌsʌl].

1st boy: Getting book and joining group. 'Oh, here's some' [ouhɪsʌm]. 'Set on big bus' [sɛdɔnbɪgbʌs]. Squeals in protest at child coming into group behind him. Now looking at picture of train. 'Go shug-shug' [gouʃʌgʃʌg].

3rd boy: 'Car.' Repeats this four times. [kɑrkɑrkɑrkaɪʌr].

1st boy: 'All fall down' [ɔfɔdaun] as he jumps off table.

4th boy: 'He took that way from me.' [hɪtʌkæweɪfʌmi].

1st girl: 'Read book' [wɪbʊk]. 'More' [mou].

1st boy: 'Get wet' [gɛdwɛt]. He is reading book again.

3rd boy: Still playing with car and truck. 'Car, truck' [kartʌ].

1st boy: 'That's mine. Bang, bang, bang' [dæsmaɪn bæŋbæŋbæŋ].

30 MONTHS
(42 children studied)

1. *Pronunciation.* The 30-monther continues to shorten or telescope words and p h r a s e s and, as at 24 months, it is usually the medial consonants which are slighted. Except for words or phrases beginning with [ð] or ending with [t], the initial and final consonant are often specific. Thus we hear 'want to' [wɔnʌ]; 'what's that' [wʌsæ], [mʌdæt], [mʌdæ], [mʌsdæ], [mʌtdæ], [mʌzæt]; 'we didn't' [wɪdn]; 'time to' [taɪmʌ]; 'another one' [nʌmʌn], [nʌdʌrwʌn]. Lisping continues with those children who have difficulty with the [s] and [ʃ] sounds. The [f] and [s] substitution for [θ] is noticeable.

When the 30-monther uses the same word several times within a few minutes, there is usually a change of pronunciation, and both consonants and vowel seem very unstable. Thus, 'house' is first [haʊt] then correctly [haʊs]; 'another' may be first [ʊnʊdʌr] then [ʊndzr]; 'cross' is perhaps [kwɔs] then [kwɑ] and [kɔs].

There is a tendency to over-pronunciation of words, or addition of sound or syllable. For example, we hear 'f l o w e r' [flɔʌwʌr], 'dog' [dɔwʌg], and 'juice' [dʒiuʌs].

2. *Voice.* The voice of the 30-monther has a firm base, but from this he ranges to extremes, sometimes to a high, strained, forced, nasalized tone, to a low, soft, almost cooing quality. The child may be using a low soft voice and suddenly it will rise to a high thin squeak if he needs something immediately. Gross motor activity is often accompanied by squealing and high pitched laughter. Quieter activity at a table, for instance, often ends with speech on a high upward inflection, a squeal or a high pitched laugh. Inflection which has been one of his best speech assets up to now, seems suddenly unstable and not well controlled. He uses a loud, emphatic, strained tone when he wants to restrain or promote action in others. Whining reaches a high point in the home and with the mother.

3. *Repetitions.* The compulsive repetition of a phrase is even more marked now than at 24 months. Most children will repeat a phrase or word occasionally, but some of them will continue interminably with m o r e force, higher pitch and volume each time. At 24 months, the repetition seemed to stem from an inner compulsion. Now it often seems to be the external stimuli which increase repetition since the child is attempting more and more to use speech as a tool to command others to his needs.

This characteristic is varied by some children who do not repeat a word or phrase at any one time, but who use the same phrase periodically within a short period often to the same person to make a personal-social contact, as 'This is my new dress,' or 'These are my shoes.'

The 30-monther also demands repetition from others. 'Do it again,' is a favorite expression, and he enjoys repetition in stories and poems, often demanding the same story day after day. One child's repetitive chant may involve the whole group as they take it up after him.

Some children tend to echo the words of an adult. The degree of this characteristic varies with the child. Developmental stuttering is usually evidenced for the first time at this age. The child who repeats a great deal will often commence to repeat just the first word or syllable of a phrase such as 'so-so I can go,' or 'Wuh-wuh-why is he doing that?' This often progresses to a tonic block at the end of this easy repetition when the child will say, 'Wuh-wuh-wuh—y is he doing that?' This block is usually broken with easy force by the child himself, and gives him no great difficulty, though it may be quite marked in his speech at this period.

4. *Relation of language and activity*. The child almost always announces his intentions before he acts, even to refinement of description, such as 'gonna make a train—gonna make a big train.' At the same time he uses speech to control a situation to his liking. At 24 months, 'No' was about the extent of his attempt at verbal control, but now he may say, 'No, this time I gon' do it—I'll do it first.' Or, 'Here, don' put it dis way, cause I can't put it in. Leave it dis way.'

He expresses his demands quite verbally as 'Want to play ball,' or 'I wanna make nuh one,' and he also commands much more easily, 'Find the ball,' 'Open the door,' 'Show me.'

5. *Language relation to others*. In the developmental examination, the child is constantly referring something to 'Mom.' He wants her to share almost everything with him: 'Lookut, Mom,' 'How you do dis, Mommie?' Sometimes he is content to look at her, or to smile at her, but he usually verbalizes to include her in the situation. He often includes the examiner in his look or smile, or with a 'show me,' he demands help from her. His commands are usually related to the adult. He seldom commands his contemporaries. As his language is becoming more accurate, he is often greatly disturbed by and protests at any inaccuracies of language in others. Instead of a 'biscuit,' he may insist that one properly call it a 'zwieback.'

6. *Tensional outlets in language situations*. Total bodily movement is the most outstanding characteristic of tensional outlet at this age, or gross movements of the head, shoulders and hands. The 30-monther usually shows a great deal of impatience during a developmental examination. He is up and down constantly, anticipating the next move. It is often difficult to get him into the room and to get him started. Some children cling to their mothers, or sit in her lap at the beginning of the examination. Once he is at the table, it is difficult to keep him there, and the examiner has to keep materials moving rapidly, for the 30-monther is not only impatient, but imperious! 'All through' [ɔfu] and 'go downstairs' [goʊdaʊnstɛ] are used constantly in an attempt to terminate the examination. He goes to the door, to the wall, to the window. At the table he may sit on it, lie down on it, put his head down, kneel on the table or crawl over it.

There is frequent lower lip protrusion. Sometimes the jaw is involved and will also protrude or shift to one side or the other. His mouth may be open a good deal of the time, and he may bite his tongue. His tongue protrudes frequently, and he may lick his lips or suck his fingers or thumb. He occasionally hunches his shoulders and he may scratch his nose, his legs, lips, or cheek, or hold his lips with his hand. Eye rubbing is frequent.

7. *Illustrative excerpts*. a. Common Expressions. 'A' [ʌ] and 'some' [sʌm] are usual prefixes to a response. 'I' [aɪ]; 'I did' [aɪdɪd]; 'I don't want to' [aɪdoʊwɔntu]; 'I don't know' [aɪoʊnoʊ]; 'I can' [aɪkæn], [aɪkʌn]; 'I can't' [aɪkænt]; 'Oh' [oʊ]; 'Lookut'

[lʊkʌt]; 'Here' [hɪ], [hɪʌ], [hɪr]; 'There' [dɛ], [dɛr]; 'Where' [ʌʌ], [wʌ], [mɛʌ]; 'How' [haʊ]; 'All through' [ɔlfu], [ɔfu].

b. Developmental Examination. Picture card: 'Bow-wow' [baʊwaʊ], 'a house' [ʌhaʊs], 'cup' [kʌp], 'a shoe' [ʌʃu], 'clock' [klɑk], 'a flag' [ʌfæg].

c. Nursery. 1st girl: Playing with clay. 'Bang, bang, bang' [bæŋ] each time as she hits clay. Hands clay to teacher. 'Cake, I making a cake' [keɪk aɪmeɪkɪŋʌkeɪk].

2nd girl: Sings as she works. 'Pop goes the weasel' [pɑpgoʊzʌwizʌl].

1st girl: Echoes the song.

2nd girl: 'A for apple' [eɪfɔrʌpl]. 'A for—a for apple' [æfɔæfɔæpʌl]. She sings this four times. 'I'm all through' [aɪmɔfru]. Repeats this three times ending with 'I'm all through everybody' [aɪmɔfruɛvribadi]. Continues to sing, 'A for apple' [eɪfɔrʌpʌl]. Note change of pronunciation.

36 MONTHS
(38 children studied)

1. *Pronunciation.* In spontaneous speech, many words and phrases are still curtailed, and the characteristics remain about as at 30 months, with the medial consonant often omitted or substituted, and the beginning and final consonant usually specific, except for words beginning with [ð]. There is, however, at 36 months, a final consonant more often present than appeared at 30 months. The sounds [θ] and [ð] are particularly noticeable at this age for the frequency of substitution for them, their omission or the general difficulty in producing t h e m. Thus, we hear, 'What's this?' [ʌsɪs], 'putting them' [pʊtɪŋʌm], 'that's all' [dæsɔl], 'what are those' [ʌʌtʌdoʊz].

With the 36-monther, there seems to be a two-way mechanism operating in his speech production. He may pronounce a word correctly, and then in a few seconds he will pronounce it incorrectly, as 'doing' [duɪŋ], [doʊɪŋ]; 'like' [laɪk], [waɪk]; 'right there' [raɪtdɛr], [waɪtdɛr]; 'that's all' [ðætsɔl], [dæsɔl]. And inversely, he may pronounce it first incorrectly and then correctly: 'ball' [bɔwʌl], [bɔl]; 'think' [sɪŋk], [θɪŋk]. And lastly, he may complete the cycle and pronounce it correctly, then incorrectly, and again correctly: 'that's all' [ðætsɔl], [dæsɔl], [ðætsɔl].

2. *Voice.* The voice of the 36-monther is, in general, of an even, normal loudness, and often in a low, soft tone. His voice seems well controlled, and though he can become commanding and emphatic, *he* seems to be in command and not the voice. When he uses a softer tone, some nasality seems to creep into the voice, while a louder, more forceful level seems to eliminate it. He has a very expressive rising inflection of surprise and pleasure. There is often a breathlessness to his pleasure and he is easily surprised. He is beginning to whisper, and often responds to whispering when other techniques fail.

3. *Repetitions.* Most children are again on an easy repetitive basis with none of the compulsion noted earlier. When, during an examination, the child does not know the answer, he will ask the question antiphonally with the examiner until she changes the question. He will repeat or echo phrases between performances, but this is not excessive. One hears, however, occasional repetition of the beginning syllable, an [ʌ] or [ʌm] is often used as a starter for speech. There are some instances of medial repetition as 'the kitty rides in-in-in that,' but tonic block on a beginning

syllable as 'I wuh——want the doll,' is quite infrequent.

4. *Relation of language and activity.* This is the high point, together with 42 months, of verbal demand for verification before proceeding with action. The child says, 'Where does it go?' 'How do you do it?' 'What do we do now?' The action is then coordinated with a verbal expression: 'There,' or 'like that.' There is a great deal of verbal demand, 'I want,' and much more verbal control of a situation.

About half the children announce their intentions before they act. With a few children activity may preclude verbal expression, but some children can talk or describe what they are doing as the activity proceeds. In the Detroit B items on the developmental examination, 'What blows?' 'What scratches?' 'What bites?' a verbal explanation will be given, usually followed by an active demonstration.

5. *Language relation to others.* Commands such as 'You build it,' 'Hey gimme,' 'You make it,' and 'Look what I made,' are the most outstanding characteristic of the 36-monther's relation to others. It is still the adult who receives most of these commands, though he can command his contemporaries when the occasion calls for it. During the developmental examination, he confirms his action or expression with the examiner by 'Don't they?' 'Isn't it?' 'Would it?' or 'Can I?' An initial concept of 'permission' from others is beginning to appear. He questions, 'How?' 'What?' 'Now what?' He invites: 'Will you do this?' During examination, he relays questions to his mother only occasionally.

6. *Tensional outlets in language situations.* At this age tongue protrusion and licking the lips seems to be the most prominent release of tension.

The 36-monther seems happier than he has been since 18 months, with his constant smiling and laughing during the examination and in the nursery, as well as in the home.

Eyes, too, afford a great release at 36 months. The child will look away from a situation which is too difficult by regarding the table, by looking upward to the ceiling, or by rolling or blinking his eyes in a short meditative interlude. Lip protrusion is frequent. Hands ands arms are in movement scratching, rubbing eyes, wiping the mouth, pulling at his clothes.

7. *Illustrative excerpts.* a. Common Expressions. 'I wanna' [aɪwɑnʌ], 'funny' [fʌnɪ], 'I'm busy' [aɪmbɪsɪ], 'I'm all through' [aɪmɔlfwu], 'I won't tell you' [aɪwoʊntɛlju], 'I don't want to' [aɪdoʊwɑnʌ], 'I can't' [aɪkænt].

b. Developmental Examination. Pictorial vocabulary: 'A auto' [ʌɔtoʊ], 'a hat' [ʌhæt], 'a telephone' [ʌtɛfoʊn], 'dat's a knife' [dætsʌnaɪf], 'dat's another hat' [dætsʌnʌrhæt], 'dat's a block' [dætsʌblɑk]. Detroit B: 'Children cries' [tʃɪldrʌnkraɪz], 'some children do' [sʌmtʃɪldrʌndu], 'some ice cream' [sʌmaɪskrim], 'the water floats' [dʌwɑtʌrfloʊts], 'the doggie growls' [dʌdɔgigraʊlz].

c. Nursery. Mike: 'Is this a gun that shoots?' [ɪzðɪsʌgʊn ætʃuts] 'Does it go bang-bang?' [dʌzʌtgoʊbæŋbæŋ]. He goes to puzzles. 'I see where that goes.' [aɪsɪmʌrðætgoʊz] Only his eyes pick out the proper piece. He continues to try and help Richie with his p u z z l e . 'Right dere, right dere' [raɪtdɛr], as he places the pieces. Richie and Mike both go to the rocker and clash. Richie tries to make Mike retreat by clapping his hands, 'No, Richie' [noʊrɪtʃi]. The boys continue to hit each other, and Mike is finally victorious. He r o c k s vigorously. Teacher says he must be careful.

'What?' [mʌʌt] he asks three times as she repeats the admonition.

Richie: Goes back to p u z z l e. 'Where's that go?' [mʌnætgoʊ]

Mike: Follows up Richie. Takes a toy iron. 'This mine' [dɪmaɪn]. He sings to himself. He irons. 'He went away' [hɪwenʌweɪ], as he points the iron at Richie. Music box is brought in. 'What's the record gonna be?' [mʌdʌrekʌrdgoʊnʌbi]

Richie: Runs to victrola. 'I wanna stand on a chair' [aɪwɑnʌstændɔnʌt-ʃeɪr].

42 Months
(20 children studied)

1. *Pronunciation.* Difficulty with [ð] which is still often substituted or omitted, and omission of the medial consonant of a word or phrase are the most outstanding characteristics of pronunciation at this age. For instance, 'I don't know' may be [aɪoʊntnoʊ] or [aɪdoʊnoʊ], and 'What's that?' is usually [mʌsæt].

There is occasional exaggeration of a word as there was at 30 months.

The pronunciation of any one word changes little in a given period except for words involving [ð].

2. *Voice.* In a group, and often in conversation with just one person, a high, full-volumed yell seems to be the normal speaking tone. The children become excited easily at this age, and it seems to be the voice which takes the lead. There is a great deal of raucous, strained quality, and the voice often breaks in an attempt to go higher and louder. Squealing and yelling are common and the 42-month group is perhaps the noisiest in the nursery. On the other hand, whispering is still a strong characteristic, and the child may whisper a request or statement, but if he is not given im-mediate response, he will yell. Thus, it is again a period of extremes of voice, but the louder extreme has the margin at 42 months.

3. *Repetitions.* Repetitions are frequent and occur with almost every child. This characteristic again has a somewhat compulsive quality as it did at 30 months, but with a slightly different emphasis. At 30 months, one can often break the repetition by introducing a new subject or object. But at 42 months, the repetition often seems to be related to another person, in demand for attention, information or encouragement. If one answers him or repeats the same phrase back to him, the repetition is usually broken and the child continues his activity, though he may have to complete the cycle and repeat just once more what he has been saying.

Developmental stuttering is again prominent and is often characterized by a tonic block on the initial syllable, the duration of which is usually longer than at 30 months. 'W——w—— why did, why—— why did you do, why did you do that?' The breathing is sometimes noticeably disturbed. It seems, however, to give the child himself no more difficulty than before. This is also the age where grimacing, cocking the head, puffing out the cheeks and similar tensional overflow appear when speech blocking occurs. In other words, more individual variations begin to appear with children whose tensional overflow affects the speech. General rate of speech seems to be faster at this period. One child's reaction to this may be to leave his sentences hanging in the air and start another without difficulty, while another child may perhaps react by blocking. The rate, at this period, may be influenced by the effort of trying to keep up with the group.

4. *Relation of language and activity*. The characteristic of verifying verbally before proceeding with action is prominent with all 42-monthers. As at 36 months, he asks 'What?' 'Where?' 'How?' beforehand, following with the activity and coordinating the activity with a verbal expression, 'This is it,' 'There,' or 'That's the way.'

He often makes running comment on what he is doing, and now after the activity is terminated, he often gives a verbal description of what he has done. We see that this is a great deal like the 36-month pattern, but there is greater refinement of description to his comment. Instead of saying, 'I did it,' or 'I made it,' he now says, 'I made a lady. This is the foot. See the l'il shoes I made.'

He still announces his intentions, and he now excuses himself from a situation by saying, 'I don't know how to write' or 'I think this is too hard,' while earlier he said, 'No, I won't,' or 'I don't want to.' He often makes judgments of his work in his running comment, 'I'm not a very good drawer,' 'I went out, didn't I?' or 'Dis is no good.'

5. *Language relation to others*. 'I want . . .' still seems the most frequent expression of the 42-monther in his relations with others. He is quite dependent upon the attention, approbation and encouragement of others, both adults and contemporaries, and he calls attention to what he is doing with 'See what I'm making.'

He needs a good deal of information and confirmation from others: 'Does this go here?' 'Does that go like this?' He continues to command the adult, 'Now you do it,' but he also commands his contemporaries with ease, 'Go away,' 'You can't,' though perhaps w i t h little social

grace! He is quite conscious of adult commands and he wants to comply, even though he often resists them. He now asks permission of both adults and contemporaries, 'Can I?' and 'Will you?'

6. *Tensional outlets in language situations*. Tongue protrusion is still prominent in release of tensional overflow. He also bites and clicks his tongue when tension is evident. His hands are prominently in movement. It should be noted here that at this age there is often a rapid and frequent shift from left to right hand activity. Voice variations are notable and characterized by whispering, sighing, squealing, laughing, chuckling, yelling, spluttering, singing, and mumbling.

7. *Illustrative excerpts*. a. Common expressions. 'What' [mʌt]; 'where' [mʌr], [mɛr]; 'how' [hau]; 'see' [si]; 'little' [lɪl]; 'funny' [fʌnɪ]; 'I want to' [aɪwanʌ], [aɪwɔnʌ]; 'I will not' [aɪwɪlnat].

b. Developmental examination. Pictorial vocabulary: 'Truck' [trʌk]; 'hat' [hæt]; 'ball' [bɔ], [bɔl]; telephone' [tɛdʌfoun]; 'airplane' [ɛrpeɪn]; 'knife' [naɪf]; 'block' [bak]; 'horse' [hɔrθ]; 'piggie' [pɪgi]; 'coat' [kout]; 'boat' [bout]; 'arm' [arm].

c. Nursery. Boy: riding bicycle. 'Git out de way' [gɪtautdʌweɪ]. Sees juice on table. 'Have we got punkin juice today?' [hævwigɔtpʌnkɪndʒustudeɪ]. Starts speech play with a girl and they throw 'witchuh' [wɪtʃʌ] back and forth several times.

2nd boy: 'I jumped right on my pants,' he says after he jumps off blocks and catches foot in his trousers. He gets on bike, 'Have to go to New York' [hævtugoutuniujɔ]. Sees napkins on table, 'Orange napkins' [andʒnæpkɪnz]. To girl, he says, 'Let me have this rattle. You know Nancy, we have pineapple juice every day.' (completely specific).

Girl: 'I want more juice' (specific).

Boy: 'I want more juice too' [aɪwɔntmourdʒusdu].

2nd boy: 'We aren't gonna rest, are we?' [wiɑrntgɑnʌrɛstɑrwi]

Girl: 'I want a cracker' (specific).

2nd girl: 'Bill, is this your chair?' (specific)

Boy: 'Here, Danny, Betty Jo's in the kitchen painting' (all specific except [kɪtsʌn]).

Girl: Goes over to prohibit playmate from bothering her construction. 'No, we're making a bridge' (specific). 'Take those over here' [tɛkdouzouvʌhɪr]. 'Did you hear what Miss Lockwood told you to do?' [dɪdjʌhɪrʍʌmɪslɑkwudtouljʌtʌdu]

48 MONTHS
(26 children studied)

1. *Pronunciation.* The child continues to omit medial sounds, with emphasis on omission of [t], [d] and [ð]. Thus, we hear, 'and that's all' [ʌnætsɔl], 'I don't want to' [aɪdouwɑnʌ], 'I don't know' [aɪountno], 'That's all' [ðæsɔl]. Any change in pronunciation in a given period occurs usually only with words containing the [ð] or [θ] sound. As with 'through,' we may hear [fru] then [θru]; or 'that's' may be [ðæts] and in a few seconds [dæs]. A child who has mastered or pronounced such sounds as [l] and [r] correctly, however, may now have a temporary relapse and use a [w] substitution. The children who have not mastered these sounds at all as yet vary in the substitutions used for them.

2. *Voice.* The four-year-old voice is beginning to subdue a bit from that of the 42-monther. However, the loud, often raucous voice quality continues with some children, especially with the boys. The 48-monther is still easily excited, especially with activity involving gross bodily movement, and the v o i c e reflects it immediately. There is some whining, and he whispers to himself. Inflection is often quite dramatic and he enjoys the drama. If he speaks of a tiny animal his voice is squeaky; if it is a steam engine, his voice is deep and husky.

3. *Repetitions.* There is little repetition at this age in comparison to some of the preceding ages. The child will repeat a phrase occasionally, but the repetition has none of the compulsive quality of the earlier ages. The child whose speech has been characterized by periods of developmental stuttering up to this time, however, may continue to have phases when repetition and blocking occur.

4. *Relation of language and activity.* The child still announces his intentions, and he usually describes what he is doing, or talks with ease while he is performing. He passes judgment more frequently on what he is doing or has done.

Speech seems to take on somewhat the same quality as a gross motor activity, for the children will throw words and phrases back and forth to one another as they throw a ball. Nonsense words are enjoyable, and there is often rhyming of nonsense words in speech play.

There is a great deal of dramatic play at this age, and when verbal and action are combined, both are often big, such as 'I threw it away, I swept it away,' while the child makes big wide gestures which conform to the feeling of the words.

There is now anticipation of future activity with verbalization. 'We'll have to wipe the table up, won't we?' Or, 'If you come to our house, I'll show you.'

He seldom asks, 'Where does that go' before placing an object. This demand for verification before acting has practically disappeared by 48 months.

5. *Language relation to others*. Demand and command are still the outstanding characteristics of speech in relation to others, and both children and adults are included. 'I wanna,' 'I don't wanna, 'Come on,' 'Put it there,' 'Sit down,' 'Go away,' 'Scram.' In demanding attention from others, he is less imperious than he was earlier. Now he may say, 'wanna see me do a funny thing?' while before he said, 'Lookut,' or 'Watch me!' He asks permission with 'Can I' or 'Can you,' and he excuses himself from a task with, 'I can't do it because I have to walk on two feet,' or 'I'm so tired, I are so worn out, I'm so worn out.'

He questions the actions of others, 'Why do you do that?' As indicated above, he enjoys speech play with others, and nonsense words are characteristic. Dramatic play is also pleasurable. One child may chant, 'I'm a witch,' and the group will respond, 'You're a witch, you're a witch,' as they all march in time to the chant.

Contact with the four-year-old sometimes seems to be lost entirely. Whether it is due to disturbed attention factors, disturbed hearing, or a combination of these or other factors, it is difficult to judge. It often seems, however, to be a real hearing difficulty. For example, one will speak to the four-year-old repeatedly without any response even though he seems to be giving attention. And inversely, he will speak to someone else repeatedly, but never hear their reply even though the volume of the response may be increased each time and he appears to be listening.

6. *Tensional outlets in language sit-uations*. Tensional overflow seems to be at a minimum during speech situations at four years. Only about half the children showed any tensional overflow such as tongue protrusion, finger in mouth, holding lower lip with teeth, lips pursed, jaw thrust forward.

7. *Illustrative excerpts*. a. Common Expressions. 'I don't know' [aɪdoʊnoʊ], [aɪoʊntnoʊ]; 'I want to' [aɪwɑnʌ]; 'I can't' (specific); 'Can I?' (specific); 'Somebody' (specific); 'Anything' (specific)[2]. It is interesting to note here the progression of expressions which the child uses in relation to self: At 24 months, he usually says 'I' or 'me'; at 36 months, he says 'you'; by 42 months, he can use 'we' and 'you'; while at 48 months, he says 'somebody' or 'anybody.'

b. Developmental Examination. Pictorial vocabulary: 'a car,' 'a hat,' 'a red cross,' 'a key,' 'an airplane,' 'a moon,' 'knife,' 'lady,' 'a coat,' 'a boat,' 'a stick,' (all specific); 'that's a flag' [ætsʌfæg], 'that's a horse' [ætsʌhɔrts].

c. Nursery. Girl: At table, 'I don't have to reach either. We'll have to wipe the table up, won't we?' (all specific). She stands to wipe off the table, and as she brushes off the crumbs, she says, 'I threw it away, I swept it away,' with large gestures (specific).

2nd girl: 'Everybody's all through except you' (specific).

3rd girl: 'Except me' (specific).

2nd girl: 'Except you' (specific). The two girls toss this back and forth several times. Now both girls go to play corner. One takes the doll carriage. 'Nancy's the daddy, I'm the mammie. I have to push it' (specific).

Boy: To second boy, 'Sit down and

---

[2] See Gesell and Ilg (2) for additional expressions.

look at the book, Freddy. Look at the fire engine, honey' [sɪtdaʊnʌnlʊkæt-ðʌbʊkfrɛdi wʊkætfaɪrendʒʌnhʌni].

3rd boy: 'Put the book up here, honey. We're going outside.' (specific except for a faint reminiscence of [θ] on the medial [s] sound).

2nd boy: Joins girls in play. 'Barbara, hi' (specific). He finds out that Barbara is the mama, and enters immediately into the spirit of the play, 'Hiyah, Mammie.'

54 MONTHS
(16 children studied)

1. *Pronunciation.* The child still has minimal difficulties in word and phrase production, but the words or phrases are not shortened or telescoped in any one place with regularity. The [ð] and [θ] still give difficulty. He may shorten words, but it seems deliberate now, and not a necessity as in 'cept' for 'except,' 'les' for 'let's,' 'rase' for 'erase.' Occasionally one hears reversals within a word such as 'bakset' for 'basket,' though it is not an outstanding characteristic.

The pronunciation of any word within a given period seldom changes except occasionally with words containing a [ð] sound or one with a medial [t].

2. *Voice.* Voice seems firm, rounded, well modulated. The child often uses a musing, contemplative tone, thinking or meditating a good deal as he talks, which gives his voice a somewhat detached quality. He often whispers to himself, carrying on quite a conversation involving two or three people and often taking all the parts himself. Highly social girls often seem to have the same inflectional tone as their mother, or as the female voice with which they come in contact most frequently.

3. *Repetitions.* He often uses [ʌm] or [ʌ] in a musing fashion at the beginning of a phrase, but he repeats seldom except for emphasis. The child who has s h o w n speech blocking earlier may again have occasional difficulty, though it has probably come and gone in a cyclic fashion since he began to show tensional outlet in his speech. If he blocks now, it is probably characterized by a slower rate, with a long breath before he starts to speak. It is perhaps the child's way of controlling or reducing the tension.

4. *Relation of language and activity.* The 48-monther had reached a stage where speech and language was a frequently employed and highly pleasurable tool. By 54 months, however, he is apparently satisfied with much less verbalization. He often goes to a task and says little. The interplay of action and verbalization is easy for him, however, and he often talks casually while performing. He may describe his activity after he has finished though it does not seem necessary to him. He seldom announces intentions, though at times when he makes an error, he may say, 'Have to 'rase it off. I made the wrong one. I'll draw it over.'

5. *Language relation to others.* The child does little commanding or demanding now unless it is to ask for information. Speech is now a more facile tool. He often judges other people and their actions. He gives a good deal of spontaneous information about what 'I can do,' and with slight stimulation will tell a long story about himself or his environment. This story may become complete improvisation and the other person may be forgotten while the story goes on indefinitely. Some children are able to cover up any inadequacy with humor or verbal banter. The child is boastful

and he likes to surprise the other person, 'You'll be surprised when you see what I'm doing,' or 'Guess what I have,' or 'You think what I have.'

Vocabulary is increasing so fast now that precision of pronunciation in others is important, for he picks up every new word, repeating it immediately and asking what it means. He often asks for several repetitions before he gets it just right.

6. *Tensional outlets in language situations.* Tongue protrusion is still a prominent tensional overflow pattern, and laughing or giggling is notable. Most of the overflow is exhibited, however, in larger activity such as standing, arm activity, wiggling in chair, moving feet.

7. *Illustrative excerpts.* a. Common Expressions. 'I don't know,' 'I said,' 'tiny,' 'surprised,' 'funny' (all specific); 'because' (specific unless it is shortened to [kɔz], 'little' ([lɪdʌl] unless it is specific).

b. Developmental Examination. 'A automobile,' 'a boy's hat,' 'a telephone,' 'key,' 'a airplane,' 'a ball,' 'knife,' 'that's a flag, red and white stripes and blue stars.' (All specific except for omission of final [d] in last phrase on 'and.')

c. Nursery. The 54-monthers were never numerous enough at any one time in the nursery to have an entire group of approximately this same age. Hence nursery conversation is omitted here.

Summary Profiles

18 Months. Somewhat quiet vocally in the nursery school unless quite disturbed. More verbalization at home with mother or at play. Long periods when activity is more important than speech. Vocalization usually combined with activity. Negative protest frequent. Good deal of jargon. Leaves off beginning and end of phrases, but makes himself understood by proper vowel and medial consonant, along with inflection. Uncertain and inconsistent in production of words; usually the vowel changes. Voice is also changeable. Experiments with voice and pitch, and has a variety of vocal overflow. Repeats syllables easily. Refers to adult for check, usually by activity. Overflow of lips, tongue, jaw, eyes and head in situation demanding attention. Smiles a great deal of the time unless disturbed. Common expressions: 'what's that?' [ʌæ], [hʌdæ], [wʌdæ]; and 'all gone' [ɔgɔ], [ɔlgɑ], [ɔlgɔn].

24 Months. Outstanding characteristic is strong repetitive, almost compulsive quality. Indications of initial syllable repetition. Seems to be consolidating past six months progress and repeats words and phrases as though fascinated. Occasionally announces his intentions before acting. Sometimes uses 'No' in attempt to control a situation, but action still quite dominant. Vowels may be inconsistent as at 18 months, but also sometimes consonants. Usually he uses beginning consonant in words and phrases, though it may be a substitution; final consonant is often present, but medial consonants slighted. In general, tone is lower and easier than at 18 months. Some nasality. Squealing and screaming still prominent. Now can ask an adult directly. Commands others occasionally. Does not need the adult for constant check. Eyes are a strong holding factor, and in situations demanding attention there is little motor overflow. Most common expressions: 'mine,' 'I want,' and 'another.'

30 Months. Speech now more a social tool, though the child is the axis. Impatience characterizes his speech and his activity. Compulsive repetition is more marked than at 24 months; he also demands repetition in verbalization and activity from others. Developmental stuttering usually evidenced here for the first time. Tensional outlets are quite outstanding and gross motor overflow is the most prominent. Tries to terminate the situation verbally. Almost always announces his intentions before he acts, even to refinement of description. Expresses demands quite verbally and commands the adult much more easily, although he seldom commands his contemporaries. L i k e s to include 'Mom' if she is near; usually does so by verbalization. Continues to shorten words and phrases, usually by slighting medial consonants. Beginnings and endings, except for beginning [ð] and ending [t], are often quite specific. Both the vowel and consonant seem unstable in pronunciation. Some over-pronunciation by addition of sound or syllable. Voice has a firm base, but varies from this to extremes. Inflection often s e e m s unstable and poorly controlled. C o m m o n expressions: 'Lookut,' 'what's that,' 'I don't want to,' 'I did,' 'I can,' 'I can't,' 'here,' 'there,' 'where,' 'how.'

36 Months. Relation of language and activity, and language relation to others is spreading in many directions. This age and 42 months are high points of verbal demand for verification before proceeding with action, which is then coordinated with a verbal expression. Commands the adult a great deal, but an initial concept of permission from others is beginning to appear. Sometimes predicts the next step in development by saying, 'Will you do this?' Shortens words and phrases as much as at 30 months, omitting or substituting medial consonant, with the initial and final consonant specific, except for [ð]. A final consonant appears more often than at 30 months. Voice is generally of an even, normal volume and often in a low, soft tone. Voice seems controlled even when commanding and emphatic. Has a very expressive rising inflection of surprise and pleasure. Whispers and often responds to whisper when other techniques fail. Shows an occasional easy repetition, although some children still show a pronounced blocking. Seems happier than any time since 18 months. Tongue and eyes offer the most release when tensional overflow is evident. Most outstanding expression: 'I wanna.'

42 Months. A high, full-volumed yell seems to be the normal speaking tone. Easily excited, and the voice seems to lead. Much raucous, strained quality, and the voice often breaks when squealing and yelling. Whispering, however, is still common. A period of extremes, with the louder the most frequent. Repetitions are frequent and of a somewhat compulsive quality, but seem related to demands for attention, information or encouragement. Developmental stuttering is again prominent. Usually verifies verbally before proceeding with action, coordinating the movement with a verbal description, and concluding with refined oral commentary of what he has done. Often comments on his own work. Quite dependent upon the attention, approbation and encouragement of others; commands with ease, but also asks permission. Most prominent characteristic: 'I want.'

48 Months. Has attained a maturity in speech which gives him freedom and pleasure. Voice is more subdued, although loud and raucous when excited. Minimal tensional overflow in speech situations. Still omits medial sounds, usually [t], [d] and [ð]. Still announces intentions and talks easily while performing. Demand and command characterize his speech. Asks permission, gives excuses, questions others' actions. Sometimes appears to have a hearing difficulty. Occasional relapse in pronunciation, especially of [l] and [r]. Common expressions: 'I wanna,' 'I don't know,' 'I can't,' 'Can I?'

54 Months. Speech has become a facile tool, but verbalization does not always seems necessary to him. Does little commanding or demanding unless to ask for information. Often judges other people and their actions. Gives a good deal of spontaneous information about what 'I can do.' May be able to cover up an inadequacy with humor or verbal banter. Boastful and likes to surprise others. Sometimes shortens words to communicate needs more rapidly. Voice seems firm, rounded, well-modulated; often uses a musing, contemplative expression. May say [ʌm] or [ʌ] at the beginning of a phrase, but seldom repeats except for emphasis. If he has shown blocking earlier, it may again appear, although he seems to have no consciousness of difficulty.

Summary

Two hundred seven children were studied in regard to the dynamics of speech production. Seven pre-school age levels from 18 to 54 months were included. No item has been included in the data presented unless the frequency warranted it. 'Voice' is necessarily based on a less objective analysis. Such a factor should be studied more carefully, and phonograph or oscillograph recordings used to make the analysis m o r e accurate. These characteristics are not 'norms,' but only an indication of some of the things in which progress can be noted and described in the speech of the child as it proceeds toward complete specificity.

No general conclusions or theoretical propositions are drawn as a result of this study. It would be of interest to investigate further such characteristics as developmental stuttering and auditory development.

It would appear that the speech therapist should be able to recognize the stage of development of the speech of any child. Better understanding of normal speech of the child will provide a clearer understanding of atypical speech.

References

1. Fisher, M. S. Language patterns of pre-school children. *Child Developm. Monogr.*, 1934, *(15)*.
2. Gesell, A. and Ilg, F. L. *Infant and Child in the Culture of Today.* New York: Harper, 1943.
3. Irwin, O. C. Infant speech: Variability and the problem of diagnosis. *JSD*, 1947, 12, 287-289.
4. McCarthy, D. *Language Development of the Pre-school Child.* Minneapolis: Univ. of Minn. Press, 1930.
5. Piaget, J. *The Language and Thought of the Child.* New York: Harcourt, Brace, 1926.
6. Smith, M. E. An investigation of the development of the sentence and the extent of vocabulary in young children. *Univ. of Iowa Studies in Child Welfare*, 1926, 3, *(5)*.
7. Wellman, B. L., Case, I. M., Mengert, I. G. and Bradbury, D. E. Speech sounds of young children. *Univ. of Iowa Studies in Child Welfare*, 1931, 5, *(2)*.
8. Williams, H. M. An analytical study of language achievement in pre-school children. *Univ. of Iowa Studies in Child Welfare*, 1937, 13, *(2)*.
9. ———. A qualitative analysis of the erroneous speech sound substitutions of pre-school children. *Univ. of Iowa Studies in Child Welfare*, 13, *(2)*.

A Disfluency Index

Fred D. Minifie

Harry S. Cooker

State University of Iowa

Verbal communication is usually defined not only in terms of the generation and transmission of speech sounds, but also in terms of the reception and detection of the information carried in these sounds. On the other hand, definitions of verbal fluency are restricted to statements about the generation and transmission of speech signals. That is, fluency refers to (a) the amount of information generated, and (b) the rate of transmission of the speech signal. Speakers who transmit a lot of information at a rather rapid rate may be described as fluent speakers. Conversely, speakers who have difficulty transmitting information, or are quite slow in transmitting that information, may be described as being more or less disfluent. The purpose of this paper is to describe a method for constructing a *disfluency* index.

Much of the early work on fluency has used words per minute (W/M) as a measurement of oral reading rate (Darley, 1940). Apparently it has been assumed that these measures of oral reading rate adequately reflected the *rate of transmission* of the speech signal. However, this method does not take into consideration the *total* number of *syllable* utterances which occur within a given reading, even though syllable rate (syllables per minute; S/M) may correspond more closely to the rate of transmission of a speech signal than does the W/M measure.

Since *words* take on distinctive *meanings* only when they are put together with other words in phrases and sentences, one might assume that the measure of words per minute, calculated in the traditional manner, more closely corresponds to the amount of information generated per unit time than it does the *rate* of transmission of the speech signal. For example, the stutterer who repeats each syllable eight or ten times does not generate much information per unit time, but might have a rather rapid rate of oral transmission. That is, he might have a rapid repetition rate when attempting each syllable.

JOURNAL OF SPEECH AND HEARING DISORDERS, 1964, Vol. 10, pp. 189-192

It is suggested that the ratio of $\frac{S}{W/M}$ be selected as an index of fluency or in this form, disfluency, in which S equals the total number of syllables uttered, and W/M equals the reading rate calculated in the traditional manner.

Comparisons between subjects on the basis of this ratio must, of course, be made using the same reading passage. Interpassage comparisons and comparisons of spontaneous speech samples are not possible since the total number of syllables and syllabic context varies from passage to passage or sample to sample. In the present study the reading rate passage from Fairbanks' *Voice and Articulation Drillbook* (1940) was used. If sufficient samples are obtained using this passage, normative data can be compiled concerning degrees of fluency impairment in the stuttering population.

In evaluating the validity of such a ratio one must consider the ways in which patterns of fluency are interrupted. It is suggested that there are two basic types of fluency interruptions. The first type might be labeled "disfluencies of syllable insertion" and includes repetitions, revisions, and interjections. The second type might be labeled "disfluencies of deliberation" and includes pauses and prolongations. Disfluencies of deliberation interrupt patterns of fluency by adding to the total amount of time required to read a given passage. Disfluencies of syllable insertion not only consume time, but also add to the total number of sounds uttered while reading a given passage.[1]

[1]It is recognized that there is considerable overlap between these two major types of fluency interrupters and that the weighting of the relative importance of each type is somewhat inconclusive.

In the face of these considerations, the ratio of $\frac{S}{W/M}$ appears to have an appropriate "face validity" in describing fluency. Consider, for example, the person whose speech behavior is characterized by disfluencies of syllable insertion. His ratio is characterized by a disproportionately large numerator which results in a large numerical disfluency index value. On the other hand, the person whose speech is characterized by disfluencies of deliberation yields a smaller denominator, which again results in a large disfluency score. Even considering the overlap between disfluencies of syllable insertion and deliberation, it appears that the method would result in a unidirectional change in the obtained fluency scores which is proportional to the amount of impairment of the fluency dimension, but relatively independent of the type of disfluent speech behavior.

Attempts to validate such an hypothesis were confined to correlational analyses. A Pearson product moment correlation coefficient of .86 was ob-

TABLE 1. Comparison of mean values of 24 college-age stutterers during Readings 1 and 5 of an adaptation sequence. Means are reported for the total number of syllables uttered (syl.), the reading rate in words per minute (W/M), and the fluency index $\left(\frac{S}{W/M}\right)$.

Reading	Syl.	W/M	$\frac{S}{W/M}$
Reading 1	240.17	143.13	2.52
Reading 5	227.67	174.65	1.77
Correlation Reading 1-5	0.92	0.86	0.99

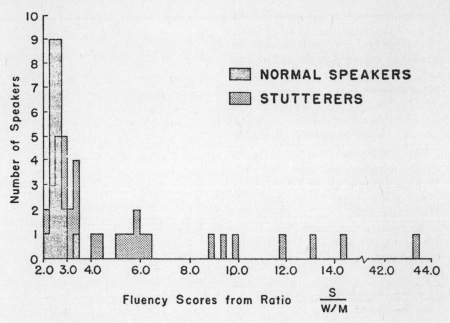

Figure 1. The distributions of fluency scores for 37 stutterers and 22 normal speakers.

tained by correlating the disfluency index ratios of 36 stutterers with mean severity ratings (obtained through direct magnitude estimation) of the same stutterers. The disfluency index correlates more highly with the severity ratings than do either the W/M (−.69) or S/M (+.72) measures. Figure 1 shows the distributions of disfluency scores for a group of stutterers and a group of normal speakers. As might be expected, several of the stutterers received disfluency scores well within the range of scores attained by normal speakers; but in general, the stutterers received much larger disfluency scores than did the normal speakers.

In order to evaluate the stability of of the disfluency index, 24 stutterers were asked to read the same passage five times, essentially completing an adaptation sequence. Table 1 shows the results of that investigation. It is noted that in Reading 5 the total number of syllables uttered is lower, the total number of W/M is greater, and the disfluency index is lower than in Reading 1. By correlating the scores on Reading 1 with the scores on Reading 5, consistency in the rank ordering of scores from Reading 1 to Reading 5 was determined. The correlations of .92 for the measure of the total number of syllables uttered, .86 for W/M, and .99 for the disfluency ratio, indicate that the disfluency ratio is the most consistent of the three measures. That is, even though the stutterers increased their general fluency performance from Reading 1 to Reading 5, they still maintained approximately the same rank order of fluency performance from Reading 1 to Reading 5.

In conclusion, it is suggested that the ratio of the total number of syllables uttered to the traditional measure of words per minute provides an effective tool for scaling fluency on a continuous dimension.

Acknowledgment

This investigation was part of a research program directed by Dr. Wendell Johnson of the University of Iowa and was supported by Grant RD-319 of the Office of Vocational Rehabilitation, Department of Health, Education, and Welfare, United States Government.

DARLEY, F. L., A normative study of oral reading rate. M.A. thesis, State Univ. Iowa, 1940.
FAIRBANKS, G., *Voice and Articulation Drillbook.* New York: Harper, 1960.

ADAPTATION AND CONSISTENCY IN THE DISFLUENT SPEECH BEHAVIOR OF YOUNG STUTTERERS AND NONSTUTTERERS

JAMES N. NEELLEY

University of Kansas, Lawrence, Kansas

ROY J. TIMMONS

Colorado State University, Fort Collins, Colorado

Sixty children, from five to eight years of age, 30 stutterers and 30 nonstutterers, were studied with regard to the adaptation and consistency phenomena of their disfluent speech behavior. A set of seven sentences was repeated five times by each subject. A frequency count of disfluent words was obtained. Neither adaptation nor consistency was an exclusive property of either experimental group. However, there was a decided tendency for the young stutterers to have the higher scores.

There is a large body of literature on adaptation and consistency in the speech of adult stutterers, but information about these phenomena in the speech of young stutterers is scant. There are apparently no published studies on adaptation in young stutterers, although Bloodstein (1960) reported the presence of consistency in the speech of a small group of children from three to six years of age. The percentage of consistency in Bloodstein's subjects varied from 50% to 100%, with an average of 77.1%. In the same article, Bloodstein described the sentence-repetition procedure that he used to measure consistency in the young nonreaders.

The purpose of the present experiment was to examine the speech of young stutterers, using a modification of Bloodstein's sentence-repetition technique, to see to what extent adaptation or consistency, or both, occur.

It was also considered important to study the speech of young nonstutterers with regard to the adaptation and consistency effects. Although these effects are supposed to be unique aspects of stuttering behavior, it was hypothesized that adaptation and consistency may be characteristic of the normal disfluencies of children considered to be nonstutterers.

JOURNAL OF SPEECH AND HEARING RESEARCH, 1967, Vol. 10, pp. 250-256.

Subjects

The subjects were 60 public school children ranging in age from five to eight years, enrolled in kindergarten, or first or second grades.

The stuttering group ($N = 30$; 23 males and 7 females) was composed of children who had been diagnosed as stutterers by their school speech clinicians. All of the children were receiving therapeutic attention, but the intensity of treatment varied from child to child.

The nonstuttering group ($N = 30$; 22 males and 8 females) consisted of children who were considered by the school clinicians to be nonstutterers. These children were selected randomly from the same classes the stuttering children attended.

Stimulus Material

The sentences used in this study were adapted in part from a subtest of the Revised Stanford-Binet Test of Intelligence (Terman and Merrill, 1937) and in part from the Bloodstein study cited earlier. The experimental sentences were as follows:

1. We are going to buy some candy bars.
2. Jack likes to feed the little puppies.
3. Tom has lots of fun playing ball.
4. We like to eat ice cream cones.
5. Jane wants to build a playhouse.
6. Fred asked his father to play with him.
7. Betty has made a dress for her doll.

The seven sentences contained a total of 51 words. With respect to word choice and length, these sentences were thought to be within the ability range of children in this study.

Procedure

Each child in the two groups was required to repeat sentences that were presented orally by an examiner. The task was standardized by employing the procedure outlined in the manual of the Revised Stanford-Binet Test of Intelligence. After an explanation of what was to be done and a brief training session, each sentence was presented to the subject, who was asked to repeat it immediately. After the seven sentences had been presented, the entire procedure was repeated four more times with the sentences always in the same order, producing a total of 35 sentences. As the subject repeated each sentence, disfluent words were marked and classified into one of the five disfluency categories by one of the authors on a printed copy of the sentences. All sessions were recorded on a Wollensak Model T-1500 tape recorder.

Analysis of the Data

Disfluent words were the basic data of the experiment. Disfluent words were defined as (1) repeated words, (2) words in which one or more syllables were repeated, (3) words in repeated phrases, (4) words containing unusually prolonged sounds, and (5) one-syllable repeated (e.g., uh-uh) interjections into the text of the experimental sentences. (Interjections such as uh-uh, although not dictionary items, were counted as words in analyzing the data.)

No count was made of the number of times a syllable, word, phrase, or interjection was repeated within an instance of disfluency; repetitions such as "ball-ball," "ball-ball-ball," "fa-father," and "fa-fa-father" were each counted as one disfluent word.

Each set of the seven sentences was referred to as "a reading."

Counting disfluent words may not be the same task as counting stuttered words. For the purposes of this study, however, it was assumed that the numerical difference between counts of "stuttered" words and counts of disfluent words in the speech of the young stuttering children would be minimal. It should be pointed out that in the studies of adult stutterers referred to later in this paper, "stuttered" words were counted and readings were used instead of sentence repetitions.

Reliability

The tape recordings made during the experiment were used to evaluate interexaminer and intraexaminer reliability in marking disfluent words. One of the authors listened twice to the recordings of three randomly selected subjects and marked the disfluent words at both listenings. The two listening sessions were separated by an interval of one week. The intraexaminer reliability, as determined by Tuthill's (1939) index of agreement, was 0.81. The interexaminer reliability of the authors on three randomly selected recordings was 0.86.

RESULTS

Disfluent Words

The mean number of disfluent words in the five readings for the stuttering group was 16.2; the standard deviation was 16.22. The mean for the nonstuttering group was 4.2 disfluent words in the five readings with a standard deviation of 5.35.

Adaptation

Although Quarrington (1959) and Tate, Cullinan, and Ahlstrand (1961) have discussed the disadvantages of adaptation percentages, they were calculated in this study. The formula used was

$$\text{Adaptation Percentage} = \left(\frac{X - Y}{X}\right)(100)$$

where X is the number of disfluent words in reading 1 and Y is the number of disfluent words in any subsequent reading.

The trends of the adaptation percentages over the five readings are described in Figure 1. A somewhat more regular adaptation trend was shown by the

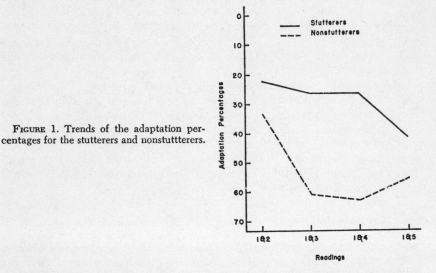

FIGURE 1. Trends of the adaptation percentages for the stutterers and nonstuttterers.

stuttering group than by the nonstuttering group. Using the trend measure described by Tate et al. (1961), the downward trend of the adaptation percentage curve for the stuttering group was significant at the 5% level; this. was not true of the curve for the nonstuttering group. The percentage of adaptation beween readings 1 and 5 for the stuttering group was not significantly different from that of the nonstuttering group.

With regard to individual adaptation performance, only three of the 30 subjects in the stuttering group had normal deviate measures of adaptation (Tate, Cullinan, and Ahlstrand, 1961) which were significant at the 5% level. None of the scores for the nonstuttering subjects was significant at the 5% level. A Mann-Whitney U computed on the distributions of these data (see Table 1) indicated, at the 5% level of confidence, that the normal deviate measures of adaptation tended to be higher in the stuttering group than in the nonstuttering group.

TABLE 1. Frequency distributions of normal deviate measures of adaptation for stutterers and nonstutterers.

Score	Stutterers	Nonstutterers
2.93 to 3.18	1°	–
2.67 to 2.92	1°	–
2.41 to 2.66	–	–
2.15 to 2.40	–	–
1.89 to 2.14	–	–
1.63 to 1.88	1°	–
1.37 to 1.62	1	1
1.11 to 1.36	3	1
0.85 to 1.10	1	1
0.69 to 0.84	8	6
0.43 to 0.68	1	–
0.17 to 0.42	1	–
−0.09 to 0.16	8	21
−0.35 to −0.10	–	–
−0.61 to −0.36	1	–
−0.87 to −0.62	–	–

°Significant at 5% level.

Consistency

Consistency percentages for contiguous readings for both groups are given in Table 2. Consistency percentages on contiguous readings were computed by the formula

$$\left(\frac{X}{Y}\right)(100)$$

where X is the number of disfluent words common to two readings and Y is the number of disfluent words in the first of the two readings. The stuttering group had significantly higher percentages of consistency than the nonstuttering group between readings 2 and 3 and between readings 3 and 4. The groups did not differ in percentages of consistency between readings 1 and 2 and readings 4 and 5.

Maximum difference consistency scores (Tate and Cullinan, 1962) were computed for individual subjects on the amount of consistency between readings 1 and 2. These scores are given in Table 3. None of the stutterers or non-

TABLE 2. Consistency percentages between specified readings for stutterers and nonstutterers.

Readings	Stutterers	Nonstutterers	t
1 and 2	40.94	23.26	1.41
2 and 3	45.45	13.79	2.69°
3 and 4	51.61	17.65	2.77°
4 and 5	46.24	37.50	0.69

°Significant at 5% level.

TABLE 3. Frequency distributions of maximum difference scores of consistency for stutterers and nonstutterers.

Score	Stutterers	Nonstutterers
9 to 10	4	–
8 to 8.9	–	–
7 to 7.9	1	1
6 to 6.9	1	–
5 to 5.9	3	1
4 to 4.9	1	2
3 to 3.9	4	1
2 to 2.9	3	1
1 to 1.9	7	6
0 to 0.9	6	18

stutterers had scores which were significant at the 5% level, although there was a tendency for the stutterers to have the higher scores.

DISCUSSION

The data show that adaptation and consistency, at least with respect to disfluent speech behavior, occur in both stuttering and nonstuttering children. However, the levels and patterning of the phenomena were somewhat different between the groups. On the individual level, it would be difficult to differentiate young stutterers from young nonstutterers on the basis of adaptation and consistency alone.

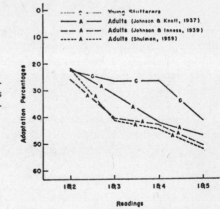

FIGURE 2. Trends of the adaptation percentages for the young stutterers of this study and for three samples of adult stutterers.

It is interesting to note in Figure 2 that the adaptation trends of the young stutterers in this study appear to be related to adaptation trends from three studies of adult stutterers (Johnson and Knott, 1937; Johnson and Inness, 1939; and Shulman, 1959). The adult stutterers, however, showed more regular and greater adaptation over five readings than did the children of this study. Only three of the normal deviate scores for the young stuttering children were significant at the 5% level, while nearly 50% of the adult stutterers in a study by Tate, Cullinan, and Ahlstrand (1961) had scores significant at that level.

Tate and Cullinan (1962) reported maximum difference scores of consistency over five readings of a 180-word passage for a group of 30 stutterers, males and females, who ranged in age from 17 to 44 years and who stuttered enough to demonstrate consistency. Nineteen of the Tate and Cullinan subjects had maximum difference scores which were significant at the 1% level. None of the 17 young stutterers who demonstrated consistency in the present study had maximum difference scores significant at the 5% level.

The data of this study indicate that the levels of adaptation and consistency in young stutterers fall between the levels for young nonstutterers and the levels for adult stutterers.

The results suggest that the adaptation and consistency in young stuttering children are early forms of the adult phenomena. Stuttering changes in several aspects as the stutterer grows older. If adaptation and consistency are aspects of stuttering, changes in adaptation and consistency scores can be anticipated. It is to be expected, then, that adaptation and consistency will have different dimensions in the speech of young stutterers and in the speech of adult stutterers. Despite the lack of significant individual consistency measures for the young stutterers described here, the relatively high frequency of consistency percentages of 50% or more may have meant that a trend toward non-chance loci of disfluencies was developing.

This report is based on a thesis submitted by Timmons to Kansas University in partial fulfillment of the requirements for the Master's degree (January, 1963). The investigation was supported partially by the Bureau of Child Research, Kansas University, and by Public Health Service Research Grant No. HD-00870, National Institute of Child Health and Development.

REFERENCES

BLOODSTEIN, O., The development of stuttering: I. Changes in nine basic features. *J. Speech Hearing Dis.*, 25, 219-237 (1960).

JOHNSON, W., and INNESS, M., Studies in the psychology of stuttering: XIII. A statistical analysis of the adaptation and consistency effects in relation to stuttering. *J. Speech Dis.*, 4, 79-86 (1939).

JOHNSON, W., and KNOTT, J., Studies in the psychology of stuttering: I. The distribution of moments of stuttering in successive readings of the same material. *J. Speech Dis.*, 2, 17-19 (1937).

SHULMAN, E., Factors influencing the variability of stuttering. In Johnson, W. (Ed.), *Stuttering in Children and Adults*. Minneapolis: Univ. Minn. Press (1959).

QUARRINGTON, B., Measures of stuttering adaptation. *J. Speech Hearing Res.*, 2, 105-112 (1959).

TATE, M. W., and CULLINAN, W. L., Measurement of consistency of stuttering. *J. Speech Hearing Res.*, 5, 272-283 (1962).

TATE, M. W., CULLINAN, W. L., and AHLSTRAND, A., Measurement of adaptation in stuttering. *J. Speech Hearing Res.*, 4, 321-339 (1961).

TERMAN, L. M., and MERRILL, M. A., *Measuring Intelligence*. Cambridge: Riverside Press (1937).

TUTHILL, C. A quantitative study of extensional meaning with special reference to stuttering. Ph.D. dissertation, State Univ. Iowa (1939).

Frequency of Syllable Repetition and 'Stutterer' Judgments

ERIC K. SANDER

'How does one enter into the category of "stutterer" and, having entered, how does one leave?' This basic question is posed by Wendell Johnson (*9*, p. 202) as a translation of the more commonly asked question, 'What is "stuttering"?' So translated, the question takes on great importance at two times in the life of an individual who stutters:

> The first of these is the moment at which the individual, usually when he is a child between two and four years of age, is looked upon for the very first time by someone, nearly always his parents, as a stutterer. . . . The other time in the life of an individual when the question ['What is "stuttering"?'] becomes crucial is when it becomes . . . , 'Am I no longer a stutterer?'

This investigation is an attempt to establish estimates of listener fluency standards for an adult speaker; it could thus be thought to concern itself with the second of the situations outlined by Johnson. Essentially, however, this research was conceived instead as a model for subsequent investigation of the child speech fluency expectations of mothers.

Van Riper (*15*, pp. 350-351) has urged that clinicians adopt the cultural norms of fluency as their criteria for distinguishing between 'primary stuttering' and 'normal' dysfluency. But information is lacking regarding the frequency with which various types of repetition or other forms of speech dysfluency must occur under differing temporal and situational conditions to elicit from most listeners a judgment of the speaker as a stutterer. In addition to theoretical implications, research information concerning the speech fluency expectations of listeners in our culture would be of interest in determining who should receive therapy, in defining treatment goals or emphases, and in establishing criteria for improvement or dismissal. If he were equipped with normative knowledge concerning not only the development of speech fluency in children (of which much is already known), but also the fluency standards of our culture (of which relatively little is known), the speech clinician could function more effectively as a counselor to parents of children who are felt to be stuttering.

Bloodstein (*2*, p. 10) writes, 'As long as listeners may differ so markedly in their definitions of defective fluency, for whatever reason, it is quite difficult to attach any absolute meaning to the term "primary stuttering."' Yet he concedes that 'it is easy enough to imagine repetitions occurring so often in a child's speech that they would alarm the great majority of parents.'

Eric K. Sander (M.A., University of Iowa, 1959) is Research Associate in Speech Pathology, Western Reserve University.

JOURNAL OF SPEECH AND HEARING DISORDERS, 1963, Vol. 28, pp. 19-30.

And clinical experience attests to many such cases.

Sound-syllable (part-word) repetition, in contrast to certain other types of speech behavior (such as interjection or revision) often classified under the more general term 'dysfluency,' is usually not present in frequent occurrence among normal-speaking children or adults. Data from the Iowa Onset Study (8, pp. 196-220) indicated that the greatest speech differences between children judged to be stutterers and those who have not acquired such reputations are in the frequency of repetition of sounds and syllables. Similar findings are reported by Johnson (7) for adult stutterers and non-stutterers. In addition, a number of recent perceptual studies using adult speakers (5, 17) suggest that sound-syllable repetitions are more often evaluated as 'stuttering' than are other types of speech dysfluency.

The number of units per repetition instance may constitute an important criterion in the minds of many listeners for differentiating 'stuttering' from 'normal' dysfluency. Among Johnson's (8) group of young stutterers the mean number of units per instance of sound-syllable repetition was 1.47 as compared with a control group mean of 1.08, a difference significant at the one per cent level. In Oxtoby's study (11) of 25 normal-speaking three-year-olds, 79 per cent of both syllable and word repetition instances consisted of but a single unit of repetition.

Often it is not meaningful in the case of adult stutterers to speak of isolated 'moments' of stuttering. In addition to their obvious speech blockages or repetitions, Wendahl and Cole (16) reported that the eight stutterers whom they studied used less rhythmical speech patterns and spoke with a greater force and strain than did normal-speaking subjects. Similarly, Van Riper (14, pp. 290-291) has observed that even in the 'normal' speech of severe stutterers the temporal patterning of syllables is broken: there are gaps, pauses, muted inflections, and unusual prolongations of normally unstressed sounds. Among allegedly stuttering preschool children, however, a disruption of rhythmic speech is much less frequently observed; indeed, the 'stutterings' themselves, usually syllable repetitions, are often unaccompanied by pronounced tension or struggle behavior.

In this investigation, basically a model for future exploration of child speech fluency standards, a three-fold question is asked: How often may an adult speaker exhibit single- (Sa-Saturday) or double- (Sa-Sa-Saturday) unit syllable repetition instances before listeners will (a) comment upon the presence of the repetitions, (b) consider the speech to be defective, and (c) classify the speaker as a stutterer?

Procedure

Speech Samples. An adult male, age 30, with normal speech, recorded a series of 24 speech samples of 100 words each, simulating without marked tension varying numbers and types of syllabic (part-word) repetitions. The classification of part-word (sound or syllable) repetition has been used by past investigators to signify anything from a prolonged block where the consonant is formed strenuously in isolation, or perhaps with a neutral vowel (k-k-kuh-keep), to a relatively effortless repetition where the initial syllable (prior to interruption) represents a duplication of the syllable in the subsequent production of the word (*kee-keep*). In this study the syllable repetitions were of the latter, essentially uneffortful type with no marked phonetic alteration.

Two types of part word syllable repetition (vowel or consonant-vowel) were employed: (a) single-unit (*Sa-Saturday*) and (b) double-unit (*Sa-Sa-Saturday*). For each of these two types of repetition, 12 speech samples of 100 words each, identical in their verbal content, were recorded; the instances of syllable repetition (single- or double-unit) in these speech samples varied from one to 15. In the first 10 speech samples (for both the single- and double-unit repetition types) the instances of syllable repetition ranged sequentially from one to 10; the last two speech samples (single- or double-unit) contained 12 and 15 repetition instances.

The speech samples with larger numbers of syllable repetitions contained the identical repetitions of the preceding samples plus the necessary additional instance(s) of syllable repetition. The loci of the repetitions were identical for both the single- and double-unit types; the repetitions were spaced rather evenly throughout the speech samples and were selected to provide a variety of consonant-vowel and vowel repetitions of the initial syllables of words. Words consisting of an isolated vowel or consonant-vowel (e.g., *to, a, be*) were spoken fluently since a syllable repetition in such an instance would also constitute a word repetition.

Listeners. Previous attempts by investigators (*1, 3, 4, 10, 13*) to define the reactions of listeners to speech dysfluency have been methodologically inhibited or handicapped by group listening procedures which inform the listener in advance of the judgments, labels, or ratings he is to make.[1] If numerous independent speech samples are to be played for the purpose of eliciting specific judgments from a group of listeners, advance instructions which may induce a preparatory perceptual bias are unavoidable. The importance of the advance instructions given to listeners has been stressed by Williams and Kent (*17*) who reported that a group of listeners instructed to mark 'stuttered' interruptions first, marked more interruptions as stuttered than they subsequently marked as normal; conversely, and not too surprisingly, listeners instructed to mark 'normal' interruptions first marked more as normal than they subsequently marked as stuttered.

Subjects for this investigation were 240 male and female college students who volunteered as listeners at the Student Union of Western Reserve University. Only one speech sample was played individually through earphones to each listener. The playback was introduced with the statement, 'Would you listen to this?' No further

[1]Berlin's (*1*) attempt to resolve the perceptual bias problem consisted of avoiding the mention of 'stuttering,' but alerting the parents to listen to each child's speech, and to list behavior that would concern them. Giolas and Williams (*6*), in their study of children's reactions to speech dysfluency, approached the perceptual bias problem obliquely; they asked each child to choose (a) the story they liked best, or (b) the speaker whom they would most like for a teacher.

comment was made. Nothing was said in advance to suggest that the experiment concerned itself with the problem of stuttering or with judgments of speech disorder. The affiliation of the experimenter with the Cleveland Hearing and Speech Center remained unknown.

At the completion of the speech playback two questions were posed orally to the listener:

1. 'How would you describe the manner of speech of the person you have just heard?'

2. 'Did you consider his speech defective?' (If so, in what way?)

Question 2 was asked following each listener's response to Question 1. Listeners were encouraged to verbalize freely; if they commented in any way about the speaker's 'hesitations,' 'nervousness,' etc., or considered his speech to be defective, a third question was asked:

3. 'Would you classify him as a stutterer?'

The above listening and questioning procedure was designed to approximate more closely than in previous research studies the types of judgments made in life situations; the instructions established, to the extent possible, a neutral or unbiased perceptual set, free from serial effect, and without the listener's foreknowledge of the subsequent judgments he was asked to make. In addition, the procedure made it possible to assess not only various dimensions of listener concern in response to the syllable repetitions, but also the listener's consciousness or awareness of the interruptions.

All listeners included in this study indicated that they had no advance knowledge from any of their friends concerning the experiment; they were advised, in turn, not to discuss the procedure with others. Responses of the listeners were recorded verbatim. The particular speech sample heard by the listener was determined by the order in which he volunteered (i.e., the first listener heard the speech sample with one instance of repetition; the second listener, the speech sample with two instances of repetition, etc.). During the first listening cycle (120 listeners) the speech samples containing the single-unit repetitions were played; the succeeding 120 listeners heard the speech samples with the double-unit repetitions. Each speech sample was heard by 10 listeners; no listener heard more than one speech sample.

Results

Awareness of Repetition. By their responses to questioning (see Table 1, pp. 27-29), the large majority of listeners indicated an awareness of the speaker's syllable repetitions. Most listeners, however, did not react to the speech samples with one or two instances of single-unit repetition. Only three of 10 listeners made some comment indicating awareness of dysfluency (e.g., 'He missed one word,' or 'He forgets and he stutters') after hearing the speech sample with one instance of single-unit syllable repetition; two of 10 listeners reacted in a similar manner (e.g., 'He gagged at one place,' or 'He started to stutter twice') to the speech sample with two instances of single-unit repetition. Comments regarding the repetitions in the remaining 10 single-unit speech samples (containing from three to 15 repetition instances) were made

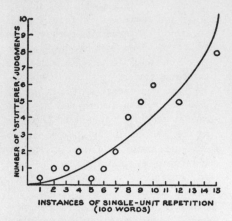

FIGURE 1. 'Stutterer' judgments of the speaker as a function of frequency of single-unit syllable repetition (120 listeners). The responses of 10 listeners are plotted for each of 12 speech samples containing from one to 15 instances of single-unit syllable repetition.

by 92 of 100 listeners. The speech sample with one instance of double-unit syllable repetition evoked responses indicating an awareness of the dysfluency (see Table 1) from seven of 10 listeners; nine of 10 listeners responded similarly to the speech sample with two instances of double-unit repetition. Thereafter the double-unit repetitions were noted, explicitly or implicitly, by all of the listeners.

'Stutterer' Judgments. Figures 1 and 2 plot the 'stutterer' judgments of listeners in relation to varying frequencies of occurrence of single- and double-unit syllable repetitions. Occasional irregularities or reversals in the number of 'stutterer' judgments with increasing syllable repetition may reflect either the small sample of listeners employed or subtle differences in dysfluent speech production from sample to sample; most likely, some combination of both factors contributed to the reversals.

In response to the single-unit repetitions (Fig. 1), the number of 'stutterer' judgments increased slowly at first, then rose more rapidly with increasing syllable repetition. The relationship, represented by a freely drawn line (Fig. 1), may be considered suggestively exponential in form. None of the speech samples containing fewer than eight instances of single-unit repetition was felt by more than two of 10 listeners to be representative of a stutterer. The repetitions were most often attributed to nervousness, loss of words, etc.

Listener responses to the double-unit repetitions (Fig. 2) indicated an early and rapid growth in the number of 'stutterer' judgments with increasing syllable repetition. The relationship suggested by a freely drawn line (Fig. 2) was parabolic. Although the speech

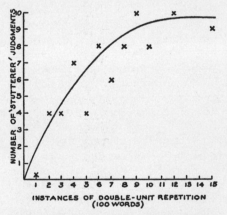

FIGURE 2. 'Stutterer' judgments of the speaker as a function of frequency of double-unit syllable repetition (120 listeners). The responses of 10 listeners are plotted for each of 12 speech samples containing from one to 15 instances of double-unit syllable repetition.

sample with only one instance of double-unit syllable repetition received no affirmative 'stutterer' judgments, four of 10 listeners felt that the speech samples with either two or three instances of double-unit repetition were spoken by stutterers. Thus, from a comparison of Figures 1 and 2, it may be seen that listeners were as likely to classify as a stutterer a speaker displaying two or three instances of double-unit repetition as one with eight instances of single-unit repetition.

Each of the speech samples with more than five instances of double-unit syllable repetition received a majority of 'stutterer' judgments. However, only at the higher frequencies of occurrence of single-unit syllable repetition (the speech samples containing 10 and 15 instances of repetition per 100 words) did a majority of listeners agree on the 'stutterer' classification. At least eight of 10 listeners were in all cases willing to classify the speaker as a stutterer if he displayed eight or more double-unit repetitions; however, only one of the single-unit speech samples, that containing 15 instances of repetition, elicited affirmative 'stutterer' judgments from eight of 10 listeners.

'Defective Speech' and 'Stutterer' Comparisons. In Figure 3 the data previously graphed in Figures 1 and 2 are grouped and a comparison is made between the number of listeners who considered the speech 'defective' and those who classified the speaker as a stutterer. Forty-one listeners felt that the speech of the speaker was defective but were unwilling for various reasons to classify him as a stutterer. Seven listeners, interestingly enough, were not

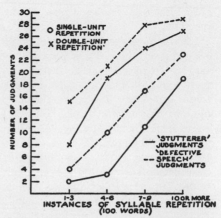

FIGURE 3. Comparison of listener responses to single- and double-unit syllable repetition instances (240 listeners). The 'stutterer' judgments of listeners are graphed along with the number of 'defective speech' judgments in relation to the frequency of occurrence for both the single- and double-unit syllable repetition instances. Data previously presented in Figures 1 and 2 are grouped.

willing to classify the speech as defective but were quite sure that the speaker was a stutterer. The remaining 192 listeners responded to both the 'defective speech' and 'stutterer' questions with consistent affirmative or negative judgments.

For single-unit repetitions, judgments of 'defective speech' increased in a linear fashion with more instances of repetition, whereas the number of 'stutterer' judgments, as noted previously, increased quite slowly initially, then rose rapidly with increases in syllable repetition. For double-unit repetitions, judgments of 'defective speech' increased rather linearly until a maximum of listener agreement was obtained, resulting in a forced leveling of the curve; 'stutterer' judgments, as previously observed, displayed a para-

129

bolic rise with increased double-unit repetition.

Listener Comments. Table 1 presents a sampling of the listeners' reactions to varying frequencies of occurrence of single- and double-unit syllable repetition instances. The most common response by far was simply, 'He stuttered,' or 'He was stuttering.' A sizable number of listeners, 29, employed the verbs 'stuttering' or 'stammering' in their descriptions of the speaker's behavior but were unwilling for various reasons (most common: 'He didn't stutter enough') to classify him as a stutterer. In context, it seemed that the term 'stuttering' was frequently used to describe heard speech repetitions or interruptions without the connotation of a speech disorder. Some listeners commented, 'He stutters because he's nervous,' 'He mainly stutters because he's not sure of what he wants to say,' etc.

Twenty-three listeners, not included as subjects in this investigation, reacted to the double-unit repetitions as 'deliberate,' 'pseudo,' or 'imitated' stuttering. These responses occurred almost entirely at the higher frequencies of double-unit repetition where a certain sense of patterned artificiality was unavoidable. Some listener reactions were: 'It seemed like it was planned; the words that he stuttered were too far between and too "well" stuttered'; 'It seemed "put on" because I would expect him to stutter on all the words with the same sound'; 'He was attempting to imitate a stutterer; there were too many articulations that were excellent and no tension or muscular problems'; etc. Only one listener commented that the single-unit repetitions sounded 'unreal' to him.

Discussion

Explanation of Repetition. When a listener under ordinary circumstances evaluates a speaker's dysfluency he is influenced by the consistency with which the speaker displays such dysfluent speech behavior over a period of time and in a number of situations. Attempts by previous researchers to force listeners to differentiate normal from abnormal speech behavior ('stuttering' from 'normal' dysfluency) on the basis of a single instance of behavior seem almost calculated to result in gross disagreement. For example, all of us may at one time move or wiggle our nose in tic-like fashion in response to local irritation (e.g., a hay-fever sufferer), or clear our throat gruffly (such behavior is not grossly different from what is sometimes classified as an 'interjection'). What determines whether such behavior is to be considered abnormal or unusually deviant? The momentary 'severity' (whatever such a term might connote) of the behavior is one consideration, but it is not necessarily the most important. The basic question is, 'Can the observer construct a plausible temporary explanation which will enable him to dismiss the subject's behavior as normal?' And, in the case of the speaker, as his syllable repetitions increase in frequency or consistency it becomes correspondingly more difficult for his listeners to invent an explanation which will leave intact his reputation as an essentially normal speaker.

The type of explanation offered by the listener for the speaker's repetitions thus appears crucial in shaping the listener's judgment of 'normal' or 'defective' speech. Bloodstein (2, p. 3) states, 'There is . . . one attribute of . . . [stuttering] which typifies it above all: the person . . . knows precisely what word he wants to say; he is simply unable for the moment to say it.' By their comments (Table 1) the listeners in this study reflected Bloodstein's observation; those who felt that the speaker 'had trouble finding words' or 'needed to get organized' were unlikely to classify him as a stutterer.

Several important variables determining listener response were left ambiguous: the type of audience, whether the subject was reading or speaking, and the speaker's familiarity with the material. Most listeners arrived at assumptions which were tacit or verbalized (see Table 1); a few listeners, however, felt that they needed more information in order to make a reliable judgment. Some of the comments were: 'Whether he is a stutterer depends on the circumstances; it could have been temporary,' 'His speech might be defective if he were familiar with the material but otherwise not,' 'He was under tension; if he was just conversing I might consider him a stutterer,' etc.

Linguistic Evolution. A few concluding thoughts are provoked by the distinction between 'stuttering' and 'stutterer.' At first glance the two terms would appear to be mutually inclusive; however, many listeners by their usage seemed to feel that it was clearly possible to 'stutter' without being a 'stutterer.' Listeners responded: 'I don't think he stuttered enough to be called a stutterer,' 'He stuttered because he couldn't find the word he wanted,' etc. In the writer's clinical experience, mothers are often unwilling to classify their child as a 'stutterer' (the term seems to connote a permanent disability), although they may speak quite freely of their child's 'stuttering.' In the language usage of listeners the term 'stuttering' need not even imply a problem that should arouse concern; laymen do not necessarily distinguish between 'stuttering' and 'normal' dysfluency, a dichotomy that has found favor among some speech pathologists.

When verbs or adjectives give birth to nouns we encounter a more severe stage of the problem. Johnson (8, p. 230) reports that once parents decide that their child is 'beginning to stutter,' a considerable time (the mean is five months) usually elapses before the judgment is made that the child has a 'speech problem.' In a provocative text, Skinner (12, p. 202) describes the evolution of trait names:

> The things to which . . . nouns refer are . . . taken to be the active causes of the aspects. We begin with 'intelligent behavior,' pass first to 'behavior which *shows* intelligence,' and then to 'behavior which *is the effect of* intelligence.'

In similar vein, it seems permissible to speak of a 'linguistic evolution' of the stuttering problem. (Reference to Table 1 provides some suggestive examples.) Borrowing Skinner's structure, we begin with 'stuttering behavior,' pass first to 'behavior which *shows* stuttering,' and then to 'behavior which occurs because the individual *is* a stutterer.' In terms of their language behavior, the responses of the listeners in this study might be grouped on a continuum beginning with 'He repeated,' or 'He hesitated' (relatively descriptive terms), passing first to 'He stuttered' (less descriptive), then to 'There was *evidence of* a speech impediment' (something removed from the behavior heard), and finally to 'He *had* a speech defect' (a 'thing-like' quality possessed by the speaker), or 'He seemed *to be* a stutterer' (a personification of the behavior).

TABLE 1. Representative comments from listeners who heard speech samples containing various frequencies of occurrence of single- or double-unit syllable repetition instances. (The first column gives the syllable repetition instances per 100 words; (S) indicates that the speaker was judged a stutterer.)

Frequency	Single-Unit Repetition	Double-Unit Repetition
1	Lucid speaker; he missed on one word.	He hesitated once, I noticed; that happens to anybody.
	Sounds like he memorized it; he forgets and he stutters.	He wasn't too easy to listen to since he stopped sometimes; he didn't seem too assured.
	Clear, slow, rather distinct.	At one time I remember he had trouble finding a word; he seemed lost for a second.
	Talked in one tone of voice; pleasing.	
2	Voice clear, pleasant; he gagged at one place.	He sounded as though he might have had a stutter (S).
	I thought he started to stutter several times—I think twice (S).	Stutters too much; wouldn't make a good public speaker (S).
	Compelling, interesting.	Sounded like a mild form of stage fright.
	Very impressing.	He stumbled on a couple of parts.
3	Very good except I noticed stuttering once or twice; may be due to nervousness.	He must at one time have had a stuttering defect.
	He could have been nervous; there were a few parts where he stuttered mildly.	He was stuttering; he stuttered three times when he first started something new; not severe (S).
	Signs of nervousness; the speech was memorized or read.	He spoke very clearly even though he did stumble over a few words.
4	He's a bit hesitant; young and inexperienced speaker.	He was just scared; he hesitated in order to think.
	A little bit mike shy because there were a few pauses that shouldn't be in there.	He stuttered, of course, but he could get by; probably wouldn't need much help, if any (S).
	He was jerky in parts which tended to destroy the fluency of it all.	He's not sure of himself; he hesitates; some of his words sort of carry over.
	He had trouble starting words (S).	He stuttered a little bit (S).
5	Sounded like he didn't know what he was saying; he hadn't prepared.	This is the case of a man who doesn't have his mind on the subject; not the sign of a real stutterer.
	He seemed to stammer every so often.	He seemed to have trouble with stuttering.

Frequency	*Single-Unit Repetition*	*Double-Unit Repetition*
	He missed a couple of words; kind of stumbled. He's reading it, but hasn't gone over it before.	His voice was very pleasant except for the couple of times he stuttered and fell over a few words (S).
6	Spoke well, but he stopped; might be nervousness that causes him to hesitate. Sometimes he's rather hesitating (S). He had a slight impediment starting the sentence; he repeated the first vowel twice.	He stuttered occasionally, but I wouldn't say badly; could be corrected with speech therapy (S). I noticed his stuttering quite a bit (S). Even when he stuttered he wasn't overtly flustered; he seemed to know that stuttering was part of his speech pattern (S).
7	Sounded like he had a slight speech defect; he would stutter slightly (S). Shy, sort of hesitant; he wasn't sure of himself or else he was scared. Stammered but was confident; he seemed to repeat the whole word instead of a letter. He seemed as if he never read it before he gave it.	He had difficulty with certain letters; otherwise his voice was pleasing (S). I wouldn't say he stuttered but he hesitated before every clause; he repeated the first syllable three times. There was the stammering that didn't always appear. He seemed to be laboring quite a bit; struggling for words as if it wasn't his natural language (S).
8	Very smooth except that he had a slight stutter (S). He's written it out, but he's learned it so well that when he pauses he forgets the right word; he's not sure of himself. Kind of broken up (S).	It was obvious he stutters (S). He was able to get across despite his speech impediment (S). He has some speech defect; faltering. There was evidence of a speech impediment (S).
9	He stutters on certain letters; he was nervous (S). I don't think he can handle short words; he has trouble with vowels. Very poor; good quality, good enunciation, but rhythm is poor (S).	If he could overcome his stuttering he would be a good speaker (S). He stuttered an awfully lot (S). I get the feeling that before he had more trouble than he has now; he could be helped with exercises (S).
10	Some stuttering; more than just hesitations when he spoke—that I know (S). He repeats his words (S). I don't think he knew his material well; very hesitant—not smooth at all; hard to listen to what he was saying for that reason.	If he hadn't stuttered he'd have been all right (S). Of course he did halt; I would say maybe he had trouble with his speech before and had some good training; it might have been worse before (S). He had an imperfection (S).
12	He stopped in the middle of some of the words and then began over again; he probably was a stutterer when he	It may be a form of stuttering—very close to it (S). He sounds as if he were reading some-

Frequency	Single-Unit Repetition	Double-Unit Repetition
	was younger and got over it.	thing he hadn't read before; he had a speech difficulty—could be a stutterer who was trying not to stutter (S).
	Spoke like an untrained person in his first stage of public speaking; traces of hesitation.	
		That he stutters makes it annoying (S).
	Unsure and unprepared. He wasn't stuttering: I got the feeling that he kept glancing at his notes; he was searching for words.	He stuttered, obviously; sounded as if he were nervous or unaccustomed to speaking; sounded like there was some kind of psychological trouble (S).
	He had sort of a stutter (S).	
15	He stuttered on the syllables (S).	He had quite a bit of trouble; he stuttered quite a bit; for the most part it was clear after he got the word out (S).
	He was slow and at times halting; he seemed to be a slight stutterer (S).	
	It was halting; I found myself listening more to his way of speech than to the content (S).	I'd call it a stutter (S).
		He goes too fast—that's why he stutters; he would need work (S).

Summary

After hearing a tape-recorded message by an adult male, 240 college subjects were interviewed concerning their reactions to the occurrence of single- (*Sa-Saturday*) or double- (*Sa-Sa-Saturday*) unit syllable repetition instances in his speech. Only one speech sample was played individually through earphones to each listener, who had no foreknowledge of the judgments he was subsequently asked to make.

The listeners were for the most part highly aware of the speaker's syllable repetitions. The single-unit syllable repetition instances were most often attributed to nervousness, loss of words, etc. Of the speech samples containing fewer than eight instances of single-unit syllable repetition (per 100 words) none was judged by more than two of 10 listeners as having been spoken by a stutterer. On the other hand, a rapid and early growth in the number of 'stutterer' judgments was observed with an increase in the frequency of occurrence of double-unit syllable repetitions. In general, a given number of double-unit syllable repetition instances evoked more 'stutterer' judgments than twice the same number of single-unit repetition instances.

Acknowledgment

Consultation by Prof. Paul H. Ptacek is acknowledged with gratitude. The author is indebted to J. Brayton Person for serving as the speaker in this investigation. Financial support was provided by the Cleveland Hearing and Speech Center.

References

1. BERLIN, C. I., Parents' diagnoses of stuttering. *J. Speech Hearing Res.*, 3, 1960, 372-379.
2. BLOODSTEIN, O., Stuttering as an anticipatory struggle reaction. In J. Eisenson (Ed.), *Stuttering: A Symposium*. New York: Harper, 1958.
3. BLOODSTEIN, O., JAEGER, W., and TUREEN, J., A study of the diagnosis of stuttering by parents of stutterers and nonstutterers. *J. Speech Hearing Dis.*, 17, 1952, 308-315.

4. BLOODSTEIN, O., and SMITH, SONJA M., A study of the diagnosis of stuttering with special reference to the sex ratio. *J. Speech Hearing Dis.*, 19, 1954, 459-466.
5. BOEHMLER, R. M., Listener responses to non-fluencies in adult speech. *J. Speech Hearing Res.*, 1, 1958, 132-141.
6. GIOLAS, T. G., and WILLIAMS, D. E., Children's reactions to nonfluencies in adult speech. *J. Speech Hearing Res.*, 1, 1958, 86-93.
7. JOHNSON, W., Measurements of oral reading and speaking rate and disfluency of adult male and female stutterers and non-stutterers. *J. Speech Hearing Dis.*, Monograph Supplement 7, June 1961, 1-20.
8. JOHNSON, W., *The Onset of Stuttering.* Minneapolis: Univ. Minnesota Press, 1959.
9. JOHNSON, W., and OTHERS, *Speech Handicapped School Children* (2nd ed.). New York: Harper, 1956.
10. MYSAK, E. D., Diagnoses of stuttering as made by adolescent boys and girls. *J. Speech Hearing Dis.*, 24, 1959, 29-33.
11. OXTOBY, E., A quantitative study of repetition in the speech of three-year-old children. Unpub. M.A. thesis, Univ. of Iowa, 1943.
12. SKINNER, B. F., *Science and Human Behavior.* New York: Macmillan, 1953.
13. TUTHILL, C. F., A quantitative study of extensional meaning with special reference to stuttering. *Speech Monog.*, 13, 1946, 81-98.
14. VAN RIPER, C., Experiments in stuttering therapy. In J. Eisenson (Ed.), *Stuttering: A Symposium.* New York: Harper, 1958.
15. VAN RIPER, C., *Speech Correction: Principles and Methods* (3rd ed.). New York: Prentice-Hall, 1954.
16. WENDAHL, R., and COLE, JANE, Identification of stuttering during relatively fluent speech. *J. Speech Hearing Res.*, 4, 1961, 281-286.
17. WILLIAMS, D. E., and KENT, LOUISE R., Listener evaluations of speech interruptions. *J. Speech Hearing Res.*, 1, 1958, 124-131.

Comments on Investigating Listener Reaction To Speech Disfluency

ERIC K. SANDER

Listener reactions have perhaps attracted more research scrutiny in the case of stuttering than for all other speech disorders combined. Such research has flourished primarily as a consequence of theories which hold the listener responsible in varying degrees for the development or the persistence of stuttering behavior. With few exceptions (Ainsworth, 1939; McDonald and Frick, 1954; Rosenberg and Curtiss, 1954), investigators of listener reaction toward stuttering or disfluent speech behavior have shunned the live interpersonal situation in favor of the control and manipulation afforded by recorded speech.[1] Perhaps mainly as a consequence of the preceding decision, researchers have also relied almost exclusively upon self-reports of listener reaction rather than upon objective behavior.

In this brief article, three methodological questions and related subquestions basic to the problem of assessing within a cognitive framework a listener's reaction toward speech disfluency will be discussed. (These are issues which become particularly important in any attempt to establish listener standards of speech fluency, as opposed, for example, to the mere comparison of listener groups.) As they are posed below, these questions may be seen to deal with: (a) listening set and speech disfluency evaluation, (b) the assumed generalization of the speech behavior, and (c) the type and extent of the listener's reaction.

1. During the listening experience, are subjects aware that they will be asked to make judgments of speech disorder? Are listeners given more than one speech sample to evaluate?

2. Are listeners told to assume that what they hear is representative of the speaker's usual behavior? Is information provided concerning the speaking situation?

3. Are the reactions of listeners

Eric K. Sander (Ph.D., Western Reserve University, 1964) is Assistant Professor of Speech Pathology at Ohio University. This article is based upon a review chapter from the author's dissertation. Gratitude is expressed for the competent guidance of Professors Paul H. Ptacek and Martin A. Young.

---

[1]Williams, et al. (1963) found that listener judgments of frequency and severity of stuttering under conditions of audiovisual observation correlated highly with auditory ratings alone; if we accept their findings, then, of course, as Luper (1959) indicates, acoustic recordings have obvious advantages over movies because of their lower cost and easier mechanical operation. But even for the preschool child whose audible behavior is accompanied by few visible signs of stuttering, representation of the total visual situation confronting him (especially elements of perceived conflict arising from the audience) may remain a potent factor in shaping a listener's judgment of the presence or absence of speech abnormality.

JOURNAL OF SPEECH AND HEARING DISORDERS, 1965, Vol. 30, pp. 159-165.

toward speech disfluency assessed solely by their assent to (or dissent from) the use of a particular label, or is a battery of questions employed? Do the assessment procedures pinpoint both the nature and intensity of a listener's reaction toward a speaker?

Listening Set and Speech Disfluency Evaluation

The effect of "set" upon perception has been well documented in the history of experimental psychology; it would need little mention in the context of assessing listener reaction toward speech disfluency save that previous investigators, excepting a minority (Giolas and Williams, 1958; Sander, 1963; Miller and Hewgill, 1964), have alerted subjects in advance of their listening experience to the possible presence of stuttering. Eager for economy, researchers have submitted groups of speech samples to assembled listener groups. Unfortunately, such a procedure dictates the practice of giving subjects prelistening knowledge of the judgments they are being asked to make; and from the standpoint of deriving basic information on speech disfluency perception one cannot disregard attendant serial effects which are probably introduced.

In an unpublished investigation by the author, the effects of three different randomly assigned prelistening instructions upon listener judgments were assessed. The listeners, 120 mothers, were interviewed mainly at supermarkets and shopping centers in the Cleveland, Ohio, area. They heard through earphones connected to a portable tape recorder one speech sample of one hundred words containing five instances of simulated single-unit syllable repetition spoken by a six-year-old boy.

Listeners in the *recall* condition were given the following instructions: "Would you listen to this recording of a little boy? Pay close attention to *what* he is saying; listen especially to the story he is telling. Afterward I will ask you questions to find out how well you listened to what the child said." Listeners in the *control* condition were simply asked: "Would you listen to this recording of a little boy?" Listeners in the *stuttering* condition were asked: "Would you listen to this recording of a little boy? Pay close attention to the *way* he is talking; listen esepecially for any signs of stuttering in his speech. Afterward I will ask you questions

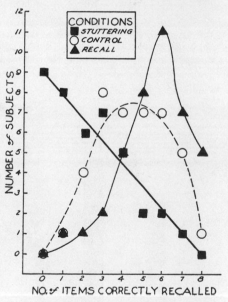

Figure 1. Mothers' recall of information spoken by a child. Eight questions were asked of each mother who had been given one of three different prelistening instructions (see text). The distribution trend for the number of items correctly recalled is represented by a broken line for the control condition, a darkened line for the stuttering condition, and a thinner line for the recall condition.

about whether the child showed any speech difficulty."

These prelistening instructions exerted a dramatic effect upon the recall of information communicated by the child. Eight questions were asked immediately after the listening experience to determine the extent of information retained. The distribution of scores graphed in Figure 1 indicated clearly that when the listeners were asked to pay close attention to the way the child was speaking they recalled very little of what he had said. Nine of the 40 mothers in the stuttering condition were unable to answer correctly any of the eight questions; the median number of correctly recalled answers was 2.0. On the other hand, the median number of questions answered correctly by mothers in the control and recall conditions was 4.5 and 5.8 respectively.

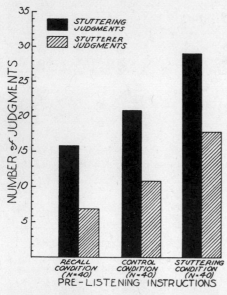

Figure 2. "Stuttering" and "stutterer" judgments of 120 mothers who had listened to a child's speech under one of three different prelistening instructions (see text).

Thus, the type of listening that occurs under a perceptual set of "trying to find stuttering" differs considerably from ordinary listening situations. Researchers must bear this fact in mind.

Evidence also strongly suggests that both the "stuttering" and "stutterer" responses of mothers are influenced by the prelistening instructions which they are given. In the study referred to in the preceding paragraph, mothers were also asked these questions: (a) Did you feel that the child was stuttering? (b) Did you feel that the child was a stutterer? Findings graphed in Figure 2 show that mothers in the stuttering condition made approximately twice as many "stuttering" and "stutterer" judgments as those in the recall condition; in the control condition, the mothers' responses fell midway between these two groups. Chi-square values of 8.70 and 7.38 for the "stuttering" and "stutterer" judgments, respectively, indicated beyond the five per cent level of confidence that these judgments were affected by the prelistening instructions.

Another study which bears on the suggestibility of listeners was carried out by Williams and Kent (1958). In separate, counterbalanced conditions they told two experimental groups of college students who listened to a contrived recording "by a person who stuttered" to mark (a) stuttered interruptions, and (b) normal interruptions. They found, not surprisingly, that the students tended to "hear" more of whatever they were instructed to mark first, at least in the cases of word and phrase repetition and interjection.

The salient point of these results is not that prelistening knowledge of the judgments to be made will invariably result in an increased number of "stuttering" or "stutterer" responses. Under differing prelistening instructions the listener might view his task as (a) deciding upon the appropriateness of a label for certain heard behavior, or (b) simply as a test of his ability to find stuttering. Let us imagine a situation in which mothers are given prelistening instructions which stress with gravity the diagnostic aspects of the term "stuttering." Under such circumstances one can also easily imagine that these mothers would be inhibited in the number of stuttering judgments which they would make. But labeling judgments aside, the listeners nevertheless would likely become more attentive to the child's speech disfluencies, and perhaps also more alarmed by them as a result of the prelistening instructions.

Assumed Generalization of the Speech Behavior

Disagreement among listeners in their responses to brief samples of speech disfluency may result from their differing assumptions concerning (a) the situation confronting the speaker, and (b) the representativeness of his displayed behavior. Researchers have curiously neglected to study the effects of situational conditions upon audience evaluations of speech disfluency; for that matter, they have failed even to specify the speaking situation in their instructions to listeners.

Pudovkin (1933, p. 140) collaborated with the Russian film theoretician, Kuleshov, to carry out an interesting experiment in film editing. They took passive close-ups of the well-known Russian actor, Mosjukhin, and joined these close-ups with other film strips in three different combinations:

In the first combination the close-up of Mosjukhin was immediately followed by a shot of a plate of soup standing on a table. It was obvious and certain that Mosjukhin was looking at this soup. In the second combination the face of Mosjukhin was joined to shots showing a coffin in which lay a dead woman. In the third the close-up was followed by a shot of a litle girl playing with a funny toy bear.

The effects of these three film strips upon an unsuspecting audience were quite astounding, according to Pudovkin:

The public raved about the acting of the artist. They pointed out the heavy pensiveness of his mood over the forgotten soup, were touched and moved by the deep sorrow with which he looked on the dead woman, and admired the light happy smile with which he surveyed the girl at play. But we knew that in all three cases the face was exactly the same.

Pudovkin's clever experiment suggests an analogy with the perception of speech disfluency. Identical recorded excerpts of speech disfluency would probably evoke divergent judgments of normality or abnormality under visually portrayed circumstances involving dissimilar degrees of perceived conflict. Few listeners, for example, would be alarmed by the speech disfluencies of an apparently frightened child reciting before a group of strangers. But these same speech disfluencies might constitute a source of worry if they occurred when the child was alone with his mother.

A listener's recognition of situational sources of disfluency is closely related to his assumption concerning the generalization of the speech behavior. Berlin (1960), alone among previous investigators, specified the generalization variable in his instructions to listeners ("If this were your child, and if this were generally the way he spoke between the ages of two and five . . ."). In contrast, researchers such as Bloodstein and Smith (1954) and Mysak (1959), both of whom used fifteen-second speech segments from allegedly nonstuttering children, have simply asked respondents to "try to judge" whether or not the children heard were stutterers. Lacking generalizational and situational information, the listener who takes such a labeling task seriously must often first decide whether the speech disfluencies he has heard are transitory or whether they reflect the child's usual speaking behavior. And so, at least in many cases, a respondent's labeling judgments may not in fact disclose his unique speech standards or disfluency tolerance; they may only mirror his best guess as to whether the child does whatever he does all of the time.

Admittedly listeners are probably incapable in any precise sense of responding to a short segment of speech disfluency *as if* it were being displayed over a considerable period of time. And from a strict behavioristic position, attempts to short-circuit an experimental analysis of behavior are difficult to justify, as Skinner (1963) convincingly argues:

> Cognitive psychologists and others still try to circumvent the explicit control of variables by describing contingencies of reinforcement to their subjects in "instructions." They also try to dispense with recording behavior in a form from which probability of response can be estimated by asking their subjects to evaluate their tendencies to respond. But a person rarely responds to a description of contingencies as he would respond under direct exposure to them, nor can he accurately predict his rate of responding, particularly the course of the subtle changes in rate which are a commonplace in the experimental analysis of behavior.

But if one cannot overcome the practical obstacles blocking an experimental analysis of behavior, failure to at least explicate the question of generalization will confound the experimental results. Of course a researcher may be interested in studying the generalization assumptions per se of listeners (as, for example, under differing situational conditions); but without generalization instructions, he cannot begin to validly relate the momentary labeling judgments with the foreseeable and more enduring action tendencies of his listeners.

Type and Extent of the Listener's Reaction

In most investigations of speech disfluency perception, listeners have been asked to make simple binary labeling choices, either (a) stuttering/not stuttering (or "normal" disfluency), or (b) stutterer/nonstutterer (or "normal" speaker). Bloodstein et al. (1952), for example, asked parents of stutterers and nonstutterers to indicate after listening to each of a series of child recordings, "whether the child just heard was a stutterer or a normal speaker." On the other hand, Berlin (1960), whose results seemingly contradict those of Bloodstein et al., grouped into a single category all those parents who used the verb "stuttering" to describe a child's speaking behavior.

At best it would seem doubtful that the unique substance of a listener's response toward speech disfluency can be fully captured merely by asking him to affirm or negate a label. Moreover, a thorough appraisal of his aggregate reaction would encompass not only the question of the judged abnormality of the behavior, but a prior assessment of the listener's awareness of the speech disfluency[2] and an exploration of its communicative effects. The listener's explanations or interpretations of the speaker's disfluencies (for example, trouble finding words, emotional disturbance, and so forth) constitute yet another dimension of his reaction. And not to be forgotten, particularly in the case of children, are the action tendencies of listeners (for example, a mother's speaking suggestions to her child).

In terms of emphasis, previous investigators have sought either to (a) ascertain the effects of carefully controlled or differentiated forms of speech disfluency upon listener reaction (Giolas and Williams, 1958; Young, 1961; Sander, 1963; Miller and Hewgill, 1964), or (b) compare the reactions toward speech disfluency of differentiated listening groups (Bloodstein et al., 1952; Mysak, 1959; Berlin, 1960). In general, excluding those investigations where listeners have been asked to count instances of stuttering, or label isolated moments of speech disfluency, a more thorough assessment of listener reaction has usually prevailed in those studies which have not sought as a primary goal to compare the reactions of two or more listening groups.

In recent studies, Giolas and Williams (1958), Sander (1963), and Miller and Hewgill (1964) have all exploited the opportunity of posing multiple questions to listeners. Giolas and Williams sought to learn whether the children react to disfluencies in adult speech; they ingeniously studied children's preferences for stories and storytellers, also noting whether the children mentioned the speech disfluencies in giving reasons for their preferences. Sander asked his 240 listeners three questions of increasing specificity: (a) How would you describe the manner of speech of the person you have just heard? (b) Did you consider his speech defective (if so, how)?, and (c) Would you classify him as a stutterer? Miller and Hewgill, who explored the effects of disfluencies upon audience ratings of speaker credibility, administered to listeners a rating instrument encompassing the dimensions of competence, trustworthiness, and dynamism.

Unfortunately, most researchers have merely asked listeners for affirmations or negations of a single labeling judgment; moreover, their methods have not allowed readers to attach clear meaning to these judgments. As an example, Bloodstein and Smith (1954) willingly sacrificed a potentially more meaningful appraisal of listener reaction (in this case, toward the speech of allegedly nonstuttering four- to six-year-olds) for the sake of their experimental design. In a footnote, these authors, who sought to relate listener reaction and perceived sex of child, state:

> The suggestion that some of the children might be stutterers was deliberately made strong in this experiment for technical reasons. With a small number of speech samples in each series there was the danger [sic] that some subjects would

---

[2] On the basis of his research, Johnson (1959, p. 230) has suggested that the perceptual reactions of roughly half of the parents in the general population are such that they fail even to "hear" the repetitions and other disfluencies in the speech of their children. But awareness of speech disfluency is not a simple construct; it may evidence itself at various levels and in varying degrees. Mothers may evince their awareness more readily on a general feeling level than on a specific analytic level. Impressions from the child's speech may be translated into personality projections; the child may, for example, be described as "shy," "embarrassed," or "nervous."

have zero diagnosis scores for both ["boy" and "girl"] series, resulting in zero difference between the two measures. . . . Since this suggestion operated equally for "boys" and "girls," and no meaning was to be attached to an absolute number of diagnoses, the strength of the suggestion was probably of little consequence otherwise.

To toss aside so lightly the question of meaning is essentially to ignore it. But the issue cannot be ignored if we wish to arrive at intelligible relationships between speech disfluency and auditor response; if choose we must, it would seem preferable to assess thoroughly (and without an induced perceptual set) a listener's reaction to one speech sample as against his slipshod evaluations of many.

Summary

In the laboratory situation the reactions of listeners toward speech disfluency are probably highly contingent upon (a) whether they are alerted prior to their listening experience to the possible presence of stuttering, and (b) their assumptions concerning the representativeness of the speaker's behavior. Researchers have tended to focus narrowly upon a listener's affirmation or denial of an isolated labeling judgment (for example, stuttering/not-stuttering, or stutterer/nonstutterer), thereby neglecting other possibly more significant (or, in any case, more easily interpreted) dimensions of auditor reaction.

References

AINSWORTH, S., Empathic breathing of auditors while listening to stuttering speech. *J. Speech Dis.*, 4, 1939, 149-156.

BERLIN, C. I., Parents' diagnoses of stuttering. *J. Speech Hearing Res.*, 3, 1960, 372-379.

BLOODSTEIN, O., JAEGER, W., and TUREEN, J., A study of the diagnosis of stuttering by parents of stutterers and non-stutterers. *J. Speech Hearing Dis.*, 17, 1952, 308-315.

BLOODSTEIN, O. and SMITH, SONJA, A study of the diagnosis of stuttering with special reference to the sex ratio. *J. Speech Hearing Dis.*, 19, 1954, 459-466.

GIOLAS, T. G. and WILLIAMS, D. E., Children's reactions to nonfluencies in adult speech. *J. Speech Hearing Res.*, 1, 1958, 86-93.

JOHNSON, W., *The Onset of Stuttering*. Minneapolis: Univ. of Minnesota Press, 1959.

LUPER, H. L., Relative severity of stuttering ratings from visual and auditory presentations of the same speech sample. *Southern Speech J.*, 25, 1959, 107-114.

McDONALD, E. T. and FRICK, J. V., Store clerks' reaction to stuttering. *J. Speech Hearing Dis.*, 19, 1954, 306-311.

MILLER, G. R. and HEWGILL, M. A., The effect of variations in nonfluency on audience ratings of source credibility. *Quarterly J. Speech*, 50, 1964, 36-44.

MYSAK, E. D., Diagnoses of stuttering as made by adolescent boys and girls. *J. Speech Hearing Dis.*, 24, 1959, 29-33.

PUDOVKIN, V. I., *Film Technique*. Enlarged edition translated and edited by I. Montagu. London: George Newnes, Ltd., 1933.

ROSENBERG, S. and CURTISS, J., The effect of stuttering on the behavior of the listener. *J. abnor. (soc.) Psychol.*, 49, 1954, 355-361.

SANDER, E. K., Frequency of syllable repetition and 'stutterer' judgments. *J. Speech Hearing Dis.*, 28, 1963, 19-30.

SKINNER, B. F., Behaviorism at fifty. *Science*, 140, 1963, 951-958.

WILLIAMS, D. E. and KENT, LOUISE, Listener evaluations of speech interruptions. *J. Speech Hearing Res.*, 1, 1958, 124-131.

WILLIAMS, D. E., WARK, MICHELLE, and MINIFIE, F. D., Ratings of stuttering by audio, visual, and audiovisual cues. *J. Speech Hearing Res.*, 6, 1963, 91-100.

YOUNG, M. A., Predicting ratings of severity of stuttering. *J. Speech Hearing Dis.*, Monograph Supplement 7, 1961, 31-54.

LOCI OF DISFLUENCIES IN THE SPEECH OF NONSTUTTERERS DURING ORAL READING

FRANKLIN H. SILVERMAN, *and* DEAN E. WILLIAMS

University of Iowa, Iowa City, Iowa

The purpose of the present study was to determine whether "disfluencies" in the speech of nonstutterers occur most frequently on words possessing the four linguistic attributes which Brown (1945) reported were related to the occurrence of "stutterings" in the speech of his stutterers. A group of 24 male nonstutterers, ranging in age from 18 to 34 years, read the same 1000-word passage used by Brown. All words judged to have been spoken disfluently, a total of 226, were analyzed for the presence of Brown's four word characteristics, i.e., initial phoneme, grammatical function, sentence position, and word length.

Disfluencies were not randomly distributed in the speech of these nonstutterers. Disfluencies occurred most frequently on words possessing the same attributes (except sentence position) as the words on which Brown reported his stutterers stuttered. The findings of this study demonstrate the essential similarity of the loci of the normal speaker's disfluencies and the stutterer's "stutterings."

Findings reported by Brown (1945) and confirmed by other investigators (Taylor, 1966) indicate that "stutterings" are not randomly distributed in the speech of stutterers, but are most likely to occur on words which: begin with consonant sounds other than /t/, /h/, /w/, and /ð/; are nouns, verbs, adverbs, or adjectives; are the first, second, or third word of a sentence; or are five letters or more in length. According to Brown, the greater the number of these four attributes a word possesses, the more likely it is to be stuttered.

Brown's findings have been cited frequently in theoretical discussions of stuttering. According to Johnson (1955), for instance, they are significant particularly for what they imply,

> . . . relative to the essential nature of stuttering behavior. The fundamental implication is that stuttering, rather than behaving like a "disorder," or "spasm," or "incoordination," or random "dyssynchronization" of the neuromuscular mechanism involved in speech, behaves like a response made to identifiable stimuli or cues with a very considerable degree of consistency or predictability (p. 16).

The results of several investigations suggest that instances of disfluency may not be distributed at random in the speech of nonstutterers. Blankenship (1964) and Maclay and Osgood (1959) have reported that instances of disfluency

JOURNAL OF SPEECH AND HEARING RESEARCH, 1967, Vol. 10, pp. 790-794.

tend to be associated with lexical rather than with function words. The category of lexical words is made up primarily of nouns, verbs, adverbs, and adjectives (Fries, 1952). The correspondence suggests that at least one of the four linguistic attributes which have been shown to influence the loci of instances of stuttering in the speech of stutterers also influences the loci of instances of disfluency in the speech of nonstutterers. No research is available concerning a relationship between the other three linguistic attributes and the loci of disfluencies of normal speakers. It is necessary to discover whether there is a positive relationship in order to determine whether researchers have been investigating a variable of stuttering behavior, per se, or have been studying, as well, a variable of the normal disfluency behavior of normal speakers.

The purpose of the present investigation was to determine whether disfluencies are randomly distributed in the speech of nonstutterers and, if not, whether they tend to occur on words possessing the same linguistic attributes as those reported by Brown (1945) and others to be related to the occurrence of stutterings in the speech of stutterers.

METHOD

Twenty-four male nonstutterers read a 1000-word passage. They were students at the University of Iowa ranging in age from 18 to 34 years with a median of 20 years. The reading passage was the 1000-word Iowa Oral Reading Test for Stutterers, Form B, Section V, the passage which was used by Brown (1945).

The speech samples were tape-recorded in a small room where the subject and the experimenter were the only persons present. The experimenter seated the subject in full view of the recording equipment, then asked him to read the passage aloud.

All words judged from the recordings to have been spoken disfluently were identified by the experimenter on copies of the reading passage. The types of disfluencies identified and the procedures used to identify them were those recommended by Johnson (1961, pp. 3-4).[1]

To obtain an estimate of the experimenter's reliability in identifying disfluent words, a self-agreement index (Sander, 1961) was obtained by comparing his original analysis of the sample from each of four subjects with analyses he made of the same samples approximately one month later. The resulting index of 0.94 indicated a level of reliability that was regarded as adequate for the purposes of this experiment.

Each word in the entire reading passage was then evaluated in terms of Brown's four linguistic attributes (Brown, 1945, p. 182). A weight of one was assigned for each of the four attributes which it possessed. The maximum possible weight per word thus was four and the minimum possible weight per

---

[1]Johnson's phrase repetition category was not used in this study since groups of words rather than single words are involved. Multiword revisions also were excluded for this reason.

word was zero. The number of words judged disfluent which possessed each weight, i.e., zero through four, was determined.

RESULTS

To permit a direct comparison between the results of this investigation and those of Brown (1945) analyses were based on populations of disfluent words rather than on subjects. Disfluent words identified in the nonstutterers' speech totaled 226. The number of disfluent words contributed by each of the 24 subjects ranged from one to 38, with a median of 7.5.

A series of proportions[2] were derived from the data reported by Brown (1945, p. 186) for his 31 stutterers, and from those of the present study. They are plotted in Figure 1. The larger the proportion, the greater was the tendency for

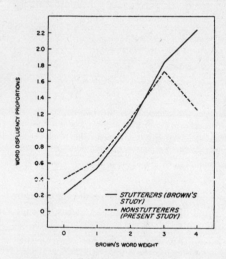

FIGURE 1. The relative proportion of the words "stuttered" by Brown's stutterers and spoken disfluently by the nonstutterers of the present study which possess each word weight. The formula which was used to compute these proportions is presented in Footnote 2.

the subjects to be disfluent on words having the specified word weight than would be expected as a result of chance. If there were no tendency for subjects in either or both of the groups to be more disfluent on words having one weight than on those having another—that is, if the instances of disfluency

---

[2]Each of these word disfluency proportions was computed by means of the following formula:

$$P_{ij} = \frac{w_{ij}/x_i}{y_{ij}/z_i} \quad (i = 1, 2; j = 0, 1, \ldots, 4)$$

where

w is the number of words which were *spoken disfluently* by the subjects in group i which possess j of Brown's four linguistic attributes.

x is the *total* number of words which were *spoken disfluently* by the subjects in group i.

y is the number of words *spoken* by the subjects in group i which possess j of Brown's four linguistic attributes (in this experiment this would be equivalent to the number of words in the reading passage which possess j of Brown's four linguistic attributes).

z is the *total* number of words which were *spoken* by the subjects in group i (in the present experiment this would be equivalent to the number of words in the reading passage).

145

were distributed at random in relation to the weights of the words with which they were associated—the proportions for the various weights all would be approximately 1.00.

Examination of Figure 1 indicates that the performance of the nonstutterers in the present study was quite similar to that of the stutterers in Brown's study (1945) on words with weights of zero, one, two, and three but was different for words with a weight of four. Specifically, they were proportionally more disfluent on words with a weight of one than they were on words with a weight of zero; more disfluent on words with a weight of two than with a weight of one; and, more disfluent on words with a weight of three than with a weight of two. They were, however, proportionally less disfluent on words with a weight

TABLE 1. The percentage of the 226 disfluent words having each of Brown's four word characteristics and the percentage of the words in the reading passage having each of the four word characteristics.

Characteristic	Percentage of Disfluent Words	Percentage in Passage
Initial phoneme	54.9	44.3
Grammatical function	82.7	63.1
Sentence position	19.5	20.7
Word length	65.0	39.2

of four than with a weight of three. Therefore, with the exception of the weight-four situation, the probability of words being spoken disfluently appears to be positively related to their weight in approximately the same degree as for the stutterers in Brown's study.

The data were analyzed further in an effort to identify factors which might account for the difference observed between Brown's stutterers and our nonstutterers at the four word weight. The percentage of the 226 disfluent words having each of Brown's four word characteristics was determined. If the subjects had a tendency to be disfluent on words possessing a given word characteristic, the percentage of disfluent words having that characteristic would be expected to exceed the percentage of the words in the reading passage possessing that characteristic. The percentage of the disfluent words possessing each of the word characteristics and the percentage of the words in the reading passage possessing each of the characteristics are presented in Table 1. The percentages of disfluent words for "initial phoneme," "grammatical function," and "word length" exceed the percentage of words possessing each of these characteristics in the reading passage. In the case of "sentence position," however, the percentage is slightly lower than that in the reading passage. This indicates that our nonstutterers were no more disfluent on the first three words of a sentence than they were on any of the other words. The fact that they are not, seems at least in part to explain the relatively small percentage of disfluent words with a weight of four in our sample as compared to the sample of stutterings upon which Brown based his analyses.

With the exception of "sentence position" (adult stutterers have relatively more difficulty "getting started" than do nonstutterers) the findings of the present study demonstrate the essential similarity of the loci of normal speaker's disfluencies and of stutterer's "stutterings."[3]

DISCUSSION

The data for this study were obtained from adult speakers. The similarity of findings between adult stutterers and nonstutterers suggests the need to pursue the same kind of investigation with children of differing age groups. There is some evidence (Bloodstein, 1960) that children may differ from adults in regard to the attributes of words on which they are disfluent.

If it is found that stuttering and nonstuttering children have similar loci of disfluency, the questions asked in research investigations must change from those asked in the past. That is, one must investigate those aspects of talking which result in predictable loci of disfluencies for both stutterers and nonstutterers. Such investigations appear to be primarily a problem for the linguist or psycholinguist. The speech pathologist should concern himself with the ways in which the loci of disfluency differ for the stutterer from that of the normal speaker.

The work reported herein was performed pursuant to a grant from the U.S. Office of Education, Department of Health, Education, and Welfare.

---

[3]To clarify whether identifying all "disfluencies" in the speech of stutterers would produce different results than identifying "stutterings," Silverman and Williams (1967) replicated Brown's study using 15 stutterers and the same classification of disfluencies used in this study of nonstutterers. Their results were in close agreement with those of Brown, indicating that one may identify "disfluencies" or "stutterings" and obtain essentially the same results.

REFERENCES

BLANKENSHIP, JANE, "Stuttering" in normal speech. *J. Speech Hearing Res.*, 7, 95-96 (1964).

BLOODSTEIN, O., The development of stuttering: II. Developmental Phases. *J. Speech Hearing Dis.*, 25, 366-376 (1960).

BROWN, S., The loci of stutterings in the speech sequence. *J. Speech Dis.*, 10, 181-192 (1945).

FRIES, C., *The Structure of English.* New York: Harcourt, Brace, & World (1952).

JOHNSON, W., The time, the place, and the problem. In Johnson, W., (Ed.), *Stuttering in Children and Adults.* Minneapolis: Univ. Minn. Press (1955).

JOHNSON, W., Measurement of oral reading and speaking rate and disfluency of adult male and female stutterers and nonstutterers. *J. Speech Hearing Dis.*, Monogr. Suppl. 7, 1-20 (1961).

MACLAY, H., and OSGOOD, C., Hesitation phenomena in spontaneous English speech. *Word* 15, 19-44 (1959).

SANDER, E., Reliability of the Iowa Speech Disfluency Test. *J. Speech Hearing Dis.*, Monogr. Suppl. 7, 21-30 (1961).

SILVERMAN, F., and WILLIAMS, D., Loci of disfluencies in the speech of stutterers. *Perceptual and Motor Skills*, 24, 1085-1086 (1967).

TAYLOR, I., What words are stuttered? *Psychol. Bull.*, 65, 233-242 (1966).

Disfluency of Normal Speakers and Reinforcement

EUGENE J. STASSI

Learning models have been used extensively to explain observables of stuttering but comparatively little use has been made of behavioral models to study disfluencies of normal speakers. Observables of stuttering have been related to learning in several ways. Among these are a comparison of stuttering adaptation to experimental extinction (8), a description of stuttering as a learned anxiety reaction because of the consistency with which stuttering follows specific cues (9), and an instrumental conditioning depiction of stuttering because of apparent operant control of amount of stuttering (2).

In the limited literature on disfluencies of normal speakers, two studies (1, 4) based on a cybernetic model (7) demonstrated that a breakdown in verbal behavior, overtly similar to stuttering, resulted from a critical time delay in auditory feedback. Stress situations also were found to produce disfluencies in the speech of normal speakers. Penalty, fear of penalty, and the requirement that an individual make and verbally express decisions about ambiguous stimuli resulted in a disorganization of verbal behavior which was similar to stuttering (3). Punishment of verbal responses has been found to

Eugene J. Stassi (M.S., Mississippi Southern College, 1960) is a Graduate Fellow in Speech Pathology and Audiology, Mississippi Southern College. This article is based on an M.S. thesis completed under the direction of Professor Robert W. Peters.

increase reaction time and has been interpreted in terms of avoidance learning and conditioned anxiety constructs (5).

Since some concepts of learning appear to relate meaningfully to stuttering phenomena, the possibility arises that, within the framework of these learning models, disfluencies may be conditioned in the speech of normal speakers.

The purpose of this study was to evaluate the effect of reward and punishment upon verbal behavior, particularly with reference to whether or not disfluencies could be elicited through negative reinforcement.

Procedure

Subjects. The subjects were 12 male and 12 female college students. All were considered normal speakers.

Verbal Task. Eight six-letter nonsense words (cycowa, uwuwid, zykave, yfegab, kixyce, udibed, koziju, ahyjyh), which were assumed to be of low associative value and within the pronouncing capabilities of the subjects, were typed in capital letters on 3″ x 5″ cards, one word to a card. The cards were arranged in the order above, remained in that order for each speaker throughout the experiment, and were turned face down before the experimental task was begun. The speaker's task was to turn one card at a time, read the word, and continue until he had read through the cards 30 times, that is, had read 30 x 8 or 240 words. He was told that after he had read each word he would be informed as to whether his pronunciation was 'right' or 'wrong.'

A 1 000 cps beep at 6 sec intervals was the signal for the speaker to turn the card and read the word. Four seconds after the beep, he heard the response of 'right' or 'wrong.' Each subject was tested alone and for each the experimental session lasted approximately half an hour.

Reinforcement Schedules. The speaker was not told that the 'right' and 'wrong' responses to his pronunciation had been programmed on magnetic tape prior to the experimental session. The responses had been recorded in a predetermined sequence as required by the experimental plan but which, of course, had no relation to the subject's pronunciation. In this sequence four different reinforcement schedules of the 'right' (reward reinforcement) and 'wrong' (punishment reinforcement) responses were used:

I. 100% reward and 0% punishment;
II. 66% reward and 33% punishment;
III. 33% reward and 66% punishment;
IV. 0% reward and 100% punishment.

Order of 'right' and 'wrong' in Schedules II and III was random. The four schedules were systematically assigned to different words for different speakers in such a way that in each speaker's total of 240 words he read 60 words under each of the four schedules. Thus, each speaker read a specified two of the eight stimulus words under a particular schedule 30 times. By the end of the experiment each word had been read under all schedules equally often by the 12 male and 12 female subjects.

The extent to which the speakers realized that the 'right' and 'wrong' responses were tape recorded on a predetermined schedule was not known. Three of the 24 speakers stated after the experimental session that they suspected that these responses were programmed on tape; however, their verbal performances did not differ from those of the other speakers. Many of the speakers apparently thought that each pronunciation was evaluated by the auditor, as evidenced by their frequent comment, 'I'm sorry,' when 'wrong' was heard following the saying of a word.

Apparatus. The directions to the subjects, the signal beep, and the 'right' and 'wrong' responses were recorded on an Ampex, Model 350, magnetic tape recorder. The pickup for the voice recordings was an Altec-Lansing, Model 21C, condenser microphone. The signal beep was produced by an audio oscillator, General Radio, Model 1302A, and the interval timing was accomplished by use of an electronic switch, Grason-Stadler, Model 829551, and an interval timer, Grason-Stadler, Model 472. The playback equipment for presentation of the material to the subjects was the Ampex recorder with an associated amplifier which fed the subjects' earphones (PDR-8 receivers). The signal level to the subjects was approximately 80 db (re .0002 d/cm²).

Measure of Disfluency. Two judges rated each word said by each subject on a nine-point scale of disfluency, where *one* represented fluency and *nine* represented extreme disfluency. Point *five* was assumed to be halfway between *one* and *nine*, the other points falling at equal distances above and below. The judges were not aware of the schedule of reinforcement. The criterion measure for each subject on each reinforcement schedule was the total score obtained by adding the ratings of the two judges for the 60 words read on that schedule. Criterion scores for each schedule thus could vary from 120 to 1 080.

Results and Discussion

Differences in the degree of judged disfluency among the four reinforcement schedules, evaluated by the Friedman two-way analysis of variance (6, pp. 166-172), were significant ($\chi_r^2 = 43.81$; $\chi_r^2{}_{.01}$ with 3 $df = 11.34$). The mean scores were 123.37, 127.41, 133.00, and 155.41 for Schedule I (100% reward and 0% punishment), II (66% reward and 33% punishment), III (33% reward and 66% punishment), and IV (0% reward and 100% punishment), respectively. Analyses using the same test were made between each possible pair among the four schedules. The schedules were significantly different beyond the 1% level, with the exception of the differences between Schedules I and II and between II and III. These χ_r^2 scores were as follows: Schedules I and II, 2.67; I and III, 10.67; I and IV, 20.17; II and III, 13.38; II and IV, 20.17; and III and IV, 20.17 ($\chi_r^2{}_{.01}$ with 1 $df = 6.64$).

A separate evaluation among schedules was made for males and females. The differences among schedules were significant for both groups (males, $\chi_r^2 = 24.93$; females, $\chi_r^2 = 24.65$; $\chi_r^2{}_{.01}$ with 3 $df = 11.34$). The mean scores for males were 123.83, 127.08, 134.25, and 160.08, and for females were 122.92,

127.75, 131.75, and 150.75 for Schedules I, II, III; and IV, respectively.

Since the mean score for the males under Schedule IV (0% reward and 100% punishment) was 160.08 as compared to 150.75 for the females under the same schedule, an evaluation was made by the Mann-Whitney U Test (6, pp. 116-127) to determine whether the two groups were significantly different in disfluency. An obtained U value of 55.5 ($U_{.01} = 42$; two-tailed test) indicated a significant difference between the two groups. A test was not made between males and females with respect to the other three conditions because differences between means were very small for the two groups under these conditions.

That the incidence of stuttering is considerably higher among males than among females is a well known fact. If this fact may be interpreted to mean that the female is less susceptible to disorganization of verbal behavior than is the male, then this susceptibility should have been reflected in the scores for the two groups of subjects. Support for this hypothesis was found only at the 100% punishment schedule (Schedule IV) where males were significantly more disfluent than females.

Three further analyses were made for evaluation of scores obtained by the subjects during the reading of the first, second, and third 80 words of the 240 words read. It was felt that perhaps disfluency occurred early in the experiment because of unfamiliarity with the task, but that it might not have persisted as the subjects became more familiar with the words. Inspection of the mean scores for the four reinforcement schedules for each 80 words indicated that there was a general decrease in amount of disfluency in time but that there was an increase in the amount of disfluency with an increase in the punishment. The mean scores were 42.71, 45.58, 47.50, and 54.08 for the first 80 pronunciations, and were 40.21, 40.75, 42.33, and 48.83 for the third 80 pronunciations. The χ_r^2 values were 22.94, 53.34, and 39.68 ($\chi_r^2{}_{.01}$ with 3 $df = 11.34$) for the first, second, and third 80 words, respectively. The trend of these values was similar to the trend obtained by the analyses for all 240 words and for males and females separately in that an increase in disfluency accompanied an increase in punishment.

The results of this study indicated that disfluencies were conditioned in the speech of normal speakers as a result of punishment of verbal behavior. The extent to which this result may be related to the development of stuttering may be only surmised; however, the behavior observed in this study does seem similar to what has been described as a learned-anxiety reaction. If an individual becomes disfluent as a result of punishment, and there is a persistence of this disfluency in response to specific word and situation cues, then it is possible that there may be some application of the results found in this study to the understanding of the onset and development of stuttering.

Summary

The effect of a predetermined schedule of reward and punishment upon the verbal behavior of normal speakers was evaluated. The subjects, 12 male and 12 female college students, read a series of nonsense words under four reinforcement schedules. Fluency-disfluency of each speaker saying each word was judged by two trained observers.

The results indicate that normal speakers become disfluent when their verbalizations are punished. Males and females were similarly affected by punishment except that males were more disfluent than females as a result of 100% punishment. The effect of reward and punishment upon verbal behavior was consistent within a short time span.

Theoretical implications concerning the onset and development of stuttering were discussed in relation to the finding that disfluencies were conditioned in the speech of normal speakers as a result of punishment.

References

1. BLACK, J. W., The effect of delayed sidetone upon vocal rate and intensity. *J. Speech Hearing Dis.*, 16, 1951, 56-60.
2. FLANAGAN, B., GOLDIAMOND, I., and AZRIN, N., Operant stuttering; the control of stuttering behavior through response, contingent consequences. *J. exp. Anal. Behav.*, 2, 1958, 173-177.
3. HILL, H. E., An experimental study of disorganization of speech and manual responses in normal subjects. *J. Speech Hearing Dis.*, 19, 1954, 295-305.
4. LEE, B. S., Artificial stutter. *J. Speech Hearing Dis.*, 16, 1951, 53-55.
5. ROTBERG, IRIS C., Effect of schedule and severity of punishment on verbal behavior. *J. exp. Psychol.*, 57, 1959, 193-200.
6. SIEGEL, S., *Nonparametric Statistics for the Behavioral Sciences*. New York: McGraw-Hill, 1956.
7. WIENER, N., *Cybernetics*. New York: Wiley, 1948.
8. WISCHNER, G. J., An experimental approach to expectancy and anxiety in stuttering behavior. *J. Speech Hearing Dis.*, 17, 1952, 139-154.
9. WISCHNER, G. J., Stuttering behavior and learning: a preliminary theoretical formulation. *J. Speech Hearing Dis.*, 15, 1950, 324-335.

DISFLUENCY BEHAVIOR OF ELEMENTARY SCHOOL STUTTERERS AND NON-STUTTERERS: THE ADAPTATION EFFECT

DEAN E. WILLIAMS *and* FRANKLIN H. SILVERMAN

University of Iowa, Iowa City, Iowa

JOSEPH A. KOOLS

University of Georgia, Athens, Georgia

A group of 184 elementary school children, 92 stutterers and 92 matched nonstutterers, performed a speaking task three times consecutively. Kindergarten and first grade children repeated a series of sentences, and the second through sixth grade children read a passage. Both the stutterers and the nonstutterers exhibited the adaptation effect. Both adapted proportionally to approximately the same degree. There was no tendency in either group for the degree of adaptation to vary as a function of grade level. Whether or not a child exhibited the adaptation effect appeared to be more closely related to how disfluent he was on his first performance of the task than to whether he had been labeled as a stutterer or a nonstutterer. Our results indictate that adaptation is not unique to stutterers, but is to be found also in normal speakers. Several implications are discussed.

Considerable research has been done on the adaptation effect in stuttering, i.e., ". . . the decrease in stuttering, as measured with reference to its frequency or severity, that occurs when a stutterer reads the same passage a number of times consecutively" (Johnson, 1955, p. 15). Numerous investigators have used the adaptation effect as support for their hypotheses about the nature of, or perpetuation of, stuttering (Brutten and Shoemaker, 1967; Eisenson, 1958; Johnson, 1967; Luper, 1954; Peins, 1961; Sheehan, 1958; Wingate, 1966; Wischner, 1950, 1952).

Stutterers used as subjects in most investigations of the adaptation effect have been adults, but two studies have been reported in which the subjects were elementary school children. The results of these two studies, one of 30 five- to eight-year-old stutterers (Neelley and Timmons, 1967) and the other of 30 ten- to thirteen-year-old stutterers (Rubin, 1957), suggest that elementary school stutterers, as a group, do exhibit the adaptation effect.

Although, traditionally, adaptation has been studied only in relation to stuttering behavior, three investigations have been reported (Brutten, 1963; Neelley and Timmons, 1967; Starbuck and Steer, 1953) in which an attempt

JOURNAL OF SPEECH AND HEARING RESEARCH, 1968
Vol. 11, pp. 622-630.

was made to determine whether normal speakers also adapt in the frequency of their speech disfluencies. This information is desirable in order to determine whether investigators have been studying a characteristic of stuttering behavior only, or a characteristic of the disfluency behavior of normal speakers as well. If normal speakers also exhibit the adaptation effect, the most probable explanation of it may be different from what it would be if this phenomenon were a unique characteristic of stuttering behavior. The results of the three studies cited suggest that normal speakers, both children and adults, do exhibit the adaptation effect. (The subjects in the Neelley and Timmons [1967] study were elementary school children, and the subjects in the other two studies were adults.) However, because of the nature of the criterion measures used, it is not possible to determine whether the normal speakers in these studies adapted proportionally to the same degree as did the stutterers.

One factor which may be of importance in determining whether an individual will exhibit the adaptation effect is the frequency of disfluency on his first performance of a task (e.g., his first reading of a passage). For adult stutterers, there is some evidence (Brutten and Shoemaker, 1967, p. 73) that the higher the individual's frequency of disfluency on his first performance of a task, the more likely he is to exhibit the adaptation effect. No data on this have been reported for elementary school children.

The questions which we will attempt to answer in this paper are:

1. Do elementary school children identified as having a stuttering problem exhibit the adaptation effect?
2. Do elementary school children with no history of a stuttering problem exhibit the adaptation effect?
3. If both groups exhibit the adaptation effect, do stutterers adapt proportionally to the same degree as do nonstutterers?
4. Does the degree of adaptation by elementary school children change as a function of age?
5. Is the probability that an elementary school child will exhibit the adaptation effect a function of the frequency of disfluency on his first performance of a task?

METHOD

Each in a group of 184 children from kindergarten through sixth grade performed a speaking task three times consecutively. Ninety-two of the children had been identified by speech clinicians and other important adults in their environment as having a stuttering problem and 92 had no history of a stuttering problem. The two groups were matched on the basis of chronological age (plus or minus six months), sex, and school grade. Mean age of the subjects in both groups was eight years and nine months, the sex ratio was approximately four males to each female, and the number of subjects from each grade in each group ranged from 11 to 16. The stutterers were referred by speech clinicians employed in one of eight programs, including six school systems, a summer camp offering speech therapy services, and the University of Iowa Speech and Hearing Clinic. All but two of the nonstutterers were from the same school system.

The kindergarten and first grade children repeated a sentence list and the second through sixth grade children read a passage three times consecutively. The list was of 10 sentences ranging in length from five to eight words. The passages read by the stutterers were approximately 100 words long and were selected from first and third grade reading books. Each nonstutterer read approximately 200 words, the paragraphs read by the stutterers plus those which immediately preceded and followed them. To minimize the influence of reading ability, the passage selected for each child was taken from a reader at least one grade below his placement at the time of experiment.

The three performances of the task by each subject were tape-recorded. On copies of the corresponding reading passage or sentence list, the experimenter identified all instances of disfluency which he heard when the recordings were played. Identified as disfluencies were part-word repetitions, word repetitions, phrase repetitions, interjections of sounds and syllables, revisions, tense pauses (tension), and disrhythmic phonations.[1] The experimenter's reliability in identifying instances of disfluency in this investigation as estimated by means of a self-agreement index (Sander, 1961) was 0.94; this value is similar to those which have been reported in other investigations (Sander, 1961).

RESULTS

Do Elementary School Children Identified as Having a Stuttering Problem Exhibit the Adaptation Effect?

The proportional adaptation measure (Silverman and Williams, 1968)— the proportion of the total number of disfluencies for all performances of the task which occur during each performance—was computed for each of the 92

---

[1]The scheme used in this study is a slightly modified version of one described by Johnson in his 1961 paper. It is based upon an unpublished revision which was completed by Johnson shortly before his death. In this revision he deleted the categories of *broken word* and *prolongation* and added the categories of *disrhythmic phonation* and *tension*. He defined these new categories as follows:

Disrhythmic phonations, identified only with words, is that kind of phonation which disturbs or distorts the so-called normal rhythm or flow of speech. The disturbance or distortion may or may not involve tension . . . and may be attributable to a prolonged sound, an accent or timing which is notably unusual, an improper stress, a break, or any other speaking-behavior infelicity not compatible with fluent speech and not included in another category. Disrhythmic phonation is a within-word category.

Tension is a disfluency phenomenon judged to exist between words, part-words, and nonwords (i.e., interjections) when at the between-point in question there are barely audible manifestations of heavy breathing or muscular tightening. The same phenomena within a word . . . would place the word in the category of *disrhythmic phonations*.

stutterers. The mean of the 92 proportions, for each of the three performances, is presented in Table 1.

TABLE 1. The mean proportion of the total disfluencies occurring during the first, second, and third performances of a task for 92 elementary school stutterers and 92 elementary school nonstutterers.

Group	Performance I	Performance II	Performance III
Stutterers	0.392	0.324	0.284
Nonstutterers	0.378	0.324	0.297

The stutterers, as a group, exhibited the adaptation effect.[2] That is, a smaller mean proportion of their total disfluencies occurred on the second performance of the task than on the first performance; and a smaller mean proportion occurred on the third performance of the task than on the second performance. Our finding for the stutterers thus agrees with those reported by other investigators.

Do Elementary School Children with No History of a Stuttering Problem Exhibit the Adaptation Effect?

The proportional adaptation measure was also computed for each of the 92 nonstutterers. The mean of the 92 proportions, for each of the three performances, is presented in Table 1.

The nonstutterers, as a group, following the same procedures as the stutterers, also exhibited the adaptation effect.[3] Our findings for the nonstutterers, thus, agree with those reported by Brutten (1963), by Neelley and Timmons (1967), and by Starbuck and Steer (1953).

Do Stutterers Adapt Proportionally to the Same Degree as Do Nonstutterers?

One of the most interesting findings of our investigation is that the nonstutterers not only showed the same trend as did the stutterers—that is, to become more fluent in successive performances of the task—but proportionally they became more fluent to approximately the same degree as did the stutter-

---

[2] A Friedman two-way analysis of variance (Siegel, 1956) was used to test the null hypothesis that in the population the proportions of the total disfluencies by each subject occurring during each of the three performances are equal. The value computed for x^2_r (i.e., 28.5) permitted the null hypothesis to be rejected at the 0.05 level of confidence.

[3] A Friedman two-way analysis of variance (Siegel, 1956) was used to test the null hypothesis that in the population the proportions of the total disfluencies by each subject occurring during each of the three performances are equal. The value computed for x^2_r (i.e., 23.0) permitted the null hypothesis to be rejected at the 0.05 level of confidence.

ers.[4] The mean proportions of disfluencies which occurred on each of the three performances of the task are very similar for the two groups of subjects (see Table 1).

The Brutten study, the Neelley and Timmons study, and the Starbuck and Steer study indicated that stutterers and nonstutterers differ in the degree to which they adapt. One reason for the differences in the findings may be a result of differences in the adaptation measures used. A characteristic shared by the adaptation measures used in these three studies, especially of the Brutten study and the Starbuck-Steer study, is that the slopes of the resulting curves are influenced by the absolute frequencies of disfluencies. The slopes of the adaptation curves obtained with the measure used in our study, on the other hand, are not influenced by group differences in numbers of disfluencies.

The data reported by Starbuck and Steer for the first three readings were reanalyzed to assess the influence of their adaptation measure (mean number of "blocks") upon the slopes of the curves for the two groups. The proportion of the total number of "blocks" reported for each of the three readings is presented for the 22 stutterers and 22 nonstutterers in Table 2. The degree of adaptation exhibited by the two groups in Table 2 is more similar than is the degree of adaptation exhibited by these same groups (on the first three readings) in Figure 1 of the Starbuck and Steer paper. Since Starbuck and Steer reported only group data, it was not possible to determine whether the differences between the stutterers and nonstutterers (Table 2) are statistically significant.

TABLE 2. Proportion of total nonfluencies occurring during the first, second, and third readings of a passage for two groups of adult subjects, 22 stutterers and 22 nonstutterers (Starbuck and Steer).

Group	Reading I	Reading II	Reading III
Stutterers	0.461	0.294	0.245
Nonstutterers	0.441	0.349	0.209

Does the Degree of Adaptation by Elementary School Children Change as a Function of Age?

The 92 elementary school stutterers and the 92 elementary school nonstutterers were divided into three grade groups: 25 kindergarten and first grade children, 31 second and third grade children, and 36 fourth, fifth, and sixth grade children. The proportion of each child's total number of disfluencies which

---

[4]The Mann-Whitney U Test (Siegel, 1956) was used to infer whether the subjects in the two groups adapt proportionally to the same degree. The test was based upon the proportions of disfluencies by each subject which occurred during the third performance of the task. The proportion of the total disfluencies for each subject occurring during the third performance was computed. The null hypothesis tested was that the proportions of the total number of disfluencies for stutterers and nonstutterers which occur during the third performance of a task are equal. The value computed for z (i.e., -0.06) was too small to permit rejection of the null hypothesis at the 0.05 level of confidence.

occurred in each performance was determined. The mean of these proportions, for each performance of the task, for each group, is presented in Table 3.

No tendency was noted for the degree of adaptation to vary systematically as a function of age for either stutterers or nonstutterers. The kindergarten and

TABLE 3. The mean proportion of the total disfluencies occurring during the first, second, and third performances of a task for six groups of elementary school children. These groups consist of 25 kindergarten and first grade stutterers, 25 kindergarten and first grade nonstutterers; 31 second and third grade stutterers, 31 second and third grade nonstutterers; and 36 fourth, fifth, and sixth grade stutterers, and 36 fourth, fifth, and sixth grade nonstutterers.

Grade Level	Group	Performance I	Performance II	Performance III
Kindergarten and First	Stutterers	0.386	0.347	0.265
	Nonstutterers	0.342	0.342	0.317
Second and Third	Stutterers	0.413	0.324	0.262
	Nonstutterers	0.364	0.318	0.318
Fourth, Fifth, and Sixth	Stutterers	0.378	0.308	0.315
	Nonstutterers	0.411	0.320	0.269

first grade, second and third grade, and fourth, fifth, and sixth grade stutterers adapted proportionally to approximately the same degree.[5] A similar conclusion was reached for the three corresponding grade groups of nonstutterers.[6]

Is the Probability that an Elementary School Child Will Exhibit the Adaptation Effect a Function of the Frequency of Disfluency on His First Performance of a Task?

The 92 elementary school stutterers and the 92 elementary school non-stutterers were divided into two groups on the basis of frequency of disfluency on the first performance of the task. Children whose frequency of disfluency was at or below their respective group median were assigned to the low frequency subgroup, and children whose frequency of disfluency was above their respective group median were assigned to the high frequency subgroup.

---

[5]The Kruskal-Wallis one-way analysis of variance (Siegel, 1956) was used to infer whether the three groups of stutterers adapt proportionally to the same degree. The test was based upon the proportions of disfluencies by each subject which occurred during the third performance of the task. The proportion of the total disfluencies for each subject occurring during the third performance was computed. The null hypothesis tested was that the proportions of the total number of disfluencies for (1) kindergarten and first grade, (2) second and third grade, and (3) fourth, fifth, and sixth grade stutterers which occur during the third performance of a task are equal. The value computed for H (i.e., 1.54) was too small to permit rejection of the null hypothesis at the 0.05 level of confidence.

[6]The Kruskal-Wallis one-way analysis of variance (Siegel, 1956) was used to infer whether the three groups of nonstutterers adapt proportionally to the same degree. The null hypothesis tested was the same as for the stutterers (see Footnote 5). The value computed for H (i.e., 2.32) was too small to permit rejection of the null hypothesis at the 0.05 level of confidence.

The 92 stutterers and the 92 nonstutterers were again divided into two groups on the basis of whether or not they exhibited the adaptation effect. A child was classified as having exhibited the adaptation effect if his third performance of the task contained a smaller proportion of his total disfluencies than did his first performance. The number of elementary school stutterers and nonstutterers in the low and high frequency subgroups who did and did not exhibit the adaptation effect is presented in Table 4.

TABLE 4. The number of kindergarten through sixth grade stutterers and nonstutterers, above (high frequency subgroup) and at or below (low frequency subgroup) their respective median disfluency frequencies on the first performance of the task, who did and did not exhibit adaptation.

Location of Score	Adaptation Exhibited	Adaptation Not Exhibited
Stutterers ($N = 92$)		
Above Median (High Frequency Subgroup)	39	9
At or Below Median (Low Frequency Subgroup)	19	25
Nonstutterers ($N = 92$)		
Above Median (High Frequency Subgroup)	37	10
At or Below Median (Low Frequency Subgroup)	17	28

The children in the high frequency subgroup exhibited the adaptation effect more frequently than did those in the low frequency subgroup.[7] This was true for both the stutterers and the nonstutterers. Whether or not a child exhibits the adaptation effect appears to be more dependent upon the frequency of disfluency on his first performance of a task than upon whether he is classified as a stutterer or a nonstutterer.

DISCUSSION

Our findings in conjunction with those of Brutten (1963), Neelley and Timmons (1967), and Starbuck and Steer (1953), indicate that adaptation is not uniquely a characteristic of the disfluency behavior of stutterers. It is a characteristic also of the disfluency behavior of normal speakers. Whether or not an individual exhibits this phenomenon appears to be more closely related to how disfluent he is on his first performance of a task than to whether he has been labeled as a stutterer or a nonstutterer.

The x^2 test for two independent samples (Siegel, 1956) was used to test the null hypothesis that children in the low frequency subgroup exhibit the adaptation effect as frequently as do those in the high frequency subgroup. The value of x^2 computed for both the stutterers (i.e., 12.69) and the nonstutterers (i.e., 14.25) was large enough to permit the null hypothesis to be rejected at the 0.05 level of confidence.

The adaptation effect has been used as evidence to support several hypotheses about the nature of, or perpetuation of, stuttering behavior. In view of the findings of our study and those previously cited, interpreting the adaptation effect as supporting certain aspects of these hypotheses may be questionable. Sheehan, for example, in discussing his fear-reduction hypothesis, interpreted the adaptation effect as follows:

> What evidence is there that the occurrence of stuttering reduces the fear which elicited the stuttering?
> Most important evidence is the existence of the adaptation effect in stuttering . . . The stuttering which occurs during the first reading decreases fear sufficiently to permit less stuttering on the second; that which occurs during the second reading reduces fear further so that there would be less stuttering on the third, etc. (Sheehan, 1958, p. 132).

Although the fact that the adaptation effect is also characteristic of the disfluency behavior of normal speakers does not disprove the fear-reduction hypothesis, the adaptation effect should not be interpreted as supporting this hypothesis unless it can be demonstrated either (1) that the adaptation effect in stutterers' and nonstutterers' speech does not arise from the same cause(s) or (2) that the adaptation effect in nonstutterers' speech is also a function of fear-reduction. The same kind of reasoning applies to other hypotheses which have been advanced, at least in part, to explain stuttering adaptation, such as "anxiety deconfirmation" (Johnson, 1967), extinction of a learned response (Wischner, 1950, 1952), "reaction inhibition" (Luper, 1954; Peins, 1961), decrease in the propositionality of the material (Eisenson, 1958; Peins, 1961), and "increasing familiarity with the prosody of the passage" (Wingate, 1966).

Since the adaptation effect does not appear to differentiate stutterers from nonstutterers, the questions asked in future investigations of this phenomenon will, of necessity, differ from those which have traditionally been asked. Rather than studying adaptation as a characteristic of the disfluency behavior of stutterers, one would investigate those aspects of talking which result in a systematic reduction in frequency of disfluency for both stutterers and nonstutterers. Such investigations may prove to be of equal or even more interest to workers in psycholinguistics than to those whose primary research interest is stuttering.

ACKNOWLEDGMENT

The project reported herein was supported by a grant from the U.S. Department of Health, Education, and Welfare, Office of Education, Division of Handicapped Children and Youth. The authors wish to express their appreciation for obtaining subjects to public school personnel in the following Iowa cities: Cedar Rapids, Davenport, Des Moines, and Solon. They also wish to express their appreciation for obtaining subjects to public school personnel in Westmoreland County, Pennsylvania, and to the staff of the University of Michigan Speech Improvement Camp (Shady Trails).

REFERENCES

BRUTTEN, E., Palmer sweat investigation of disfluency and expectancy adaptation. *J. Speech Hearing Res.*, 6, 40-48 (1963).

BRUTTEN, E., and SHOEMAKER, D., *The Modification of Stuttering*. Englewood Cliffs, New Jersey: Prentice-Hall (1967).

EISENSON, J., A perseverative theory of stuttering. In Jon Eisenson (Ed.), *Stuttering: A Symposium*. New York: Harper, 223-272 (1958).

JOHNSON, W., The time, the place, and the problem. In Wendell Johnson (Ed.), *Stuttering in Children and Adults*. Minneapolis: Univ. Minn. Press, 3-24 (1955).

JOHNSON, W., Measurement of oral reading and speaking rate and disfluency of adult male and female stutterers and nonstutterers. *J. Speech Hearing Dis.*, Monogr. Suppl. 7, 1-20 (1961).

JOHNSON, W., Stuttering. In Wendell Johnson and Dorothy Moeller (Eds.), *Speech Handicapped School Children* (3rd ed.). New York: Harper & Row, 229-329 (1967).

LUPER, H., The consistency of selected aspects of behavior in the repetitions of stuttered words. Ph.D. dissertation, Ohio State Univ. (1954).

NEELEY, J., and TIMMONS, R., Adaptation and consistency in the disfluent speech behavior of young stutterers and nonstutterers. *J. Speech Hearing Res.*, 10, 250-256 (1967).

PEINS, MARYANN, Adaptation effect and spontaneous recovery in stuttering expectancy. *J. Speech Hearing Res.*, 4, 91-99 (1961).

RUBIN, M., A study of the consistency and adaptation effects in ten to thirteen-year-old stutterers. M.A. thesis, Brooklyn College (1957).

SANDER, E., Reliability of the Iowa Speech Disfluency Test. *J. Speech Hearing Dis.*, Monogr. Suppl. 7, 21-30 (1961).

SHEEHAN, J., Conflict theory of stuttering. In Jon Eisenson (Ed.), *Stuttering: A Symposium*. New York: Harper, 121-166 (1958).

SIEGEL, S., *Nonparametric Statistics for the Behavioral Sciences*. New York: McGraw-Hill (1956).

SILVERMAN, F., and WILLIAMS, D., A proportional measure of stuttering adaptation. *J. Speech Hearing Res.*, 11, 444-446 (1968).

STARBUCK, H., and STEER, M., The adaptation effect in stuttering speech behavior and in normal speech behavior. *J. Speech Hearing Dis.*, 18, 252-255 (1953).

WINGATE, M., Prosody in stuttering adaptation. *J. Speech Hearing Res.*, 9, 550-556 (1966).

WISCHNER, G., Stuttering behavior and learning: a preliminary theoretical formulation. *J. Speech Hearing Dis.*, 15, 324-335 (1950).

WISCHNER, G., An experimental approach to expectancy and anxiety in stuttering. *J. Speech Hearing Dis.*, 17, 139-154 (1952).

Listener Evaluations
Of Speech Interruptions

Dean E. Williams

Louise R. Kent

Certain kinds of interruptions which occur in normal speech are often not discernible from those popularly considered to constitute stuttering. The assumption, however, that individuals are able to discriminate consistently between 'stuttered' and 'n o r m a l' speech interruptions is still commonly accepted. This is expressed explicitly by West (*4*) in the statement, '. . . everyone but the expert knows what *stuttering* is.' This assumption has been sustained in spite of an accumulation of evidence to the contrary (*1, 2, 3*).

The present study was designed to test the following hypothesis: Individuals do not *consistently* respond to interruptions in speech as either stuttered or normal. The specific problem was to determine whether individuals are more likely to classify interruptions as 'stuttered' when instructed to listen for stuttered interruptions and, conversely, more likely to classify the same interruptions as 'normal' when instructed to listen for normal interruptions.

Dean E. Williams, (Ph.D., State University of Iowa, 1952) is Assistant Professor of Speech and Theatre, Speech and Hearing Clinic, Indiana University. Louise R. Kent, (M.A., Indiana University, 1957) is currently in private practice in Baton Rouge, Louisiana.

JOURNAL OF SPEECH AND HEARING RESEARCH, 1958, Vol. 1, pp. 124-131.

Stimulus Material

The stimulus material was a 900-word tape-recorded s p e e c h. The speech contained 52 speech interruptions distributed among six types of nonfluencies as follows: syllable repetition — one-syllable (3), two-syllable (3) and three-syllable (4); prolongations (9); interjections (13); word repetitions (4); phrase repetitions (5); revisions (11). The syllable repetitions consisted of one, two and three repetitions of the initial syllable of words. Only syllables beginning with consonant sounds were included and no particular sounds appeared more frequently than any other. Of the nine prolongations, lasting one second each, six were in the initial position of words and three were in the medial position of words; no sound was duplicated. The interjections were 'er' and 'ah'; four occurred at the end of phrases, one at the end of a sentence and eight between words. Word and phrase repetitions should be self-explanatory. The revisions w e r e divided three, six and two, in the initial, medial and final positions of sentences, respectively.

The recorded voice was that of a normal speaker with a clinical knowledge of speech correction. A casual, conversational style of delivery was simulated; the speaker avoided noticeable changes in reading rate and inflection in order to make the contrived interruptions appear as natural as possible. Criterion judgments were obtained from three trained speech correctionists.

In order to test the assumption that the stimulus material was not clearly discriminable as either stuttered or non-stuttered speech, 32 subjects (15 males and 17 females) in introductory public speaking classes who did not participate in the experiment proper were asked to listen to the speech. These subjects were instructed to judge it according to a rating sheet ordinarily used by the instructor in rating the speeches of students in public speaking classes. The students were also instructed to record on the rating sheets their personal impression of the speech and the speaker along with any criticisms or comments. These students were told that the speaker was a person in an introductory public speaking class; that is, they were *not* told that the speaker stuttered.

The ratings made by the students were on such qualities as organization, interest, grammar, articulation and vocabulary, and are not of particular interest to this study. The comments, however, are of interest. Fourteen of the students used the word 'stuttering' or 'stammering' in their comments; five mentioned 'speech defect,' but not 'stuttering'; and 13 made no reference to speech defects.

Some of the comments made by those students who mentioned no speech defect are interesting in that they represent a variety of reactions to the speech. Abstracts from these comments are as follows:

Body (of speech) was confusing and poorly organized.

Dull.

He was sort of a George Gobel type speaker.

Was it the speaker's purpose to slur some of his words?

His time and articulation was rather poor.

His words are in too much of a monotone.

His speech wasn't well learned.

He is not sure of his speech.

Sounds like 'Just Plain Bill' after taxes.

His voice was raspy and distracting.

It sounded like a poor job of memorizing.

It was concluded that the speech nonfluencies inserted into the recorded speech were (1) sufficiently obvious to attract the attention of many observers and (2) not deviant to the extent that the speaker was evaluated as a stutterer by more than one-half of the observers.

Procedure

A total of 70 subjects (38 males and 32 females) were used in the experiment proper. Group I was composed of 36 subjects (22 males and 14 females), while Group II was comprised of 34 subjects (16 males and 18 females). These subjects were recruited from freshman and sophomore classes at Indiana University; no subjects had received training in speech correction.

Subjects in the two experimental groups were told that they would hear a recorded speech given by a person who *stuttered*. Each subject was provided with a mimeographed copy of the speech; no indication of the speech interruptions appeared on this copy. Both groups were instructed to follow the speech on their copies as they listened to the recording and to mark through the words or spaces between

TABLE 1. Actual versus obtained percentage distribution of types of interruptions marked under instructions to mark *all* interruptions.

Categories of Interruptions	Percentage Distribution		
	Actual Stimulus Material	Obtained Group I	Group II
TOTAL	100.0*	93.7*	94.2*
Syllable repetition			
One-syllable	5.8	5.4	5.3
Two-syllable	5.8	5.7	5.7
Three-syllable	7.7	7.7	7.6
Prolongations	17.3	17.1	16.9
Interjections	25.0	20.9	21.5
Word repetitions	7.7	7.3	7.2
Phrase repetitions	9.6	9.3	9.3
Revisions	21.1	20.3	20 7

*Based on actual total of 52 interruptions.

words where they heard interruptions. This procedure was repeated three times for each group under three sets of instructions.

When the record was played for the first time to Group I, the instructions were to mark the *stuttered* interruptions. The papers were then collected and new sheets distributed. When the recording was played the second time, the instructions were to mark *all* interruptions. The papers were again collected and new sheets distributed. The instructions given before the recording was played for the third time were to mark the *normal* interruptions.

For Group II the order of instructions was reversed. The subjects were instructed first to mark *normal* interruptions, second to mark *all* interruptions and third to mark *stuttered* interruptions.

Before the record was played for the first time for either group, the experimenter pointed out that in the normal course of speaking, interruptions may be, and frequently are,

uttered which do not necessarily denote stuttering. It was emphasized that there were no right nor wrong answers, that the papers would not be graded in any way, that subjects need not put their names on the papers and that the purpose of the study would be defeated if the subjects copied from each other. The subjects were instructed not to mark pauses.

The middle or second condition in which the subjects of both groups were instructed to mark *all* interruptions was essentially a control condition used to determine whether the groups differed as to the number of interruptions responded to as such. The subjects in Group I responded on the average to 93.7% of the total of 52 interruptions and subjects in Group II responded on the average to 94.2% of the total.

In Table 1 the actual percentage distribution of the different types of interruptions inserted in the stimulus material are compared with the percentage distributions obtained from the two groups under instructions to

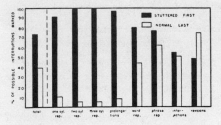

FIGURE 1. Percent of possible interruptions marked on eight categories by *Group I*, which marked stuttered interruptions first, normal last.

mark *all* interruptions. It is clear that the subjects in both groups responded at frequencies closely approximating the actual relative frequencies of the types of interruptions inserted into the speech. The results also reflect favorably upon the fidelity of the recording.

Results

The responses from the two groups of subjects yielded data corresponding to the two sets of instructions: (a) mark the stuttered interruptions and (b) mark the normal speech interruptions.

The mean number of times that a particular type of interruption was marked was computed separately un-

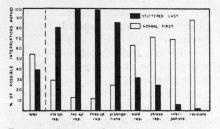

FIGURE 2. Percent of possible interruptions, marked on eight categories by *Group II*, which marked normal interruptions first, stuttered last.

der the two sets of instructions for both groups. For each type of interruption, four means were obtained: 1. that for Group I under instructions to mark stuttering, 2. that for Group I under instructions to mark normal interruptions, 3. that for Group II under instructions to mark normal interruptions and 4. that for Group II under instructions to mark stuttering. Since the number of interruptions in the stimulus material varied from one type of interruption to another, the obtained means were converted to percent of interruptions possible of a given type. For example, when instructed to mark stuttered interruptions, Group I marked a mean number of 8.7 instances of prolongations. There were actually 9 instances of prolongations in the stimulus material; the subjects responded to 96.6% of the total possible. These data are presented in Figures 1 and 2.

Inspection of Figures 1 and 2 reveals that the order of instructions introduced a bias. Group I, instructed first to mark stuttered interruptions, classified more interruptions as stuttered than they subsequently marked as normal; and conversely, Group II, instructed to mark normal interruptions first, classified more interruptions as normal than they subsequently marked as stuttered. The bias is most clearly demonstrated in the categories of word repetition, phrase repetition and interjections. Group I, marking stuttered interruptions first, classified more interruptions in these categories as stuttered than as normal; while Group II, marking normal interruptions first, classified more of them as normal than as stuttered. The bias, although discernible, was much less marked in the categories of revisions, syllable repetitions and prolongations. In these categories the two groups were in relative agreement *in spite of* the bias introduced by the order of instructions. Revisions were primarily considered normal interruptions while syllable repetitions and prolongations were primarily considered as stuttering.

The procedure used in this study allowed the subjects to reverse their judgments. Under instruction to mark stuttered interruptions, a subject might mark a particular interruption as 'stuttered,' and later under instruction to mark normal interruptions, might judge the same interruption to be 'normal.'

The number of instances of inconsistent responses on each category of interruption was tabulated for each group. Then, for each group, these numbers were divided by the total number of responses made in the corresponding category under (a) instructions to mark stuttered interruptions and (b) instructions to mark normal interruptions. The quotients obtained represent a ratio between the *total* number of responses made in a particular category (under one or the other set of instructions) and the *number of inconsistent responses* made in this same category. This ratio is termed an *Index of Confusion* because it is employed as a measure of the

degree of confusion of the subjects as to whether a particular type of interruption should be judged stuttered or normal.

An example of the computational procedure used is as follows. The subjects in Group I, when instructed to mark stuttered interruptions, classified 193 instances of revisions as stuttering. When asked to mark normal interruptions, they reversed judgment on 138 of these instances. There were, then, 138 inconsistent responses in the category of revisions. Here the Index of Confusion is 71.5, which is interpreted to indicate a high degree of confusion on the part of the subjects in Group I as to whether revisions should be classified as stuttered interruptions. The Indexes of Confusion for the two

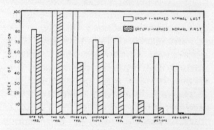

FIGURE 4. Indexes of confusion on eight categories of interruptions when subjects were instructed to mark *normal* interruptions.

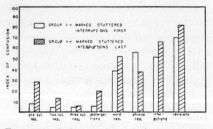

FIGURE 3. Indexes of confusion on eight categories of interruptions when subjects were instructed to mark *stuttered* interruptions.

groups are presented in Figures 3 and 4. The results of the analysis of inconsistent responses support and complement the data depicted in Figures 1 and 2. Figure 3 shows that when subjects were instructed to mark stuttered interruptions, they evidenced less confusion on the categories of syllable repetitions and prolongations than on the categories of revisions, interjections, word repetitions and phrase repetitions; hence, the subjects were more positive that syllable repetitions and prolongations were stuttered interruptions and less positive on revisions, interjections, word repetitions and phrase repetitions.

Figure 4 shows that when subjects were instructed to mark normal interruptions, they evidenced less confusion on revisions, interjections, phrase repetitions and word repetitions than on syllable repetitions and prolongations; hence, the subjects were more positive that revisions, interjections, phrase repetitions and word repetitions were representative of normal speech and less positive on syllable repetitions and prolongations. Thus, confusion or inconsistency, although varying in degree, existed on all categories of interruptions regardless of the order of instructions.

In considering these inconsistency data, it is important to be aware again of the bias introduced by the order of instructions. Inconsistency was greater for Group I when marking normal interruptions and greater for Group II when marking stuttered interruptions. The bias apparently operated in the following fashion: Group I initially classified a large proportion of the interruptions as stuttering; therefore, a large number of the interruptions subsequently judged to be normal had previously been marked as stuttering, thus increasing Group I's Index of Confusion under instructions to mark normal interruptions. Group II, on the other hand, initially classified a large proportion of the interruptions as normal; therefore, a large number of the interruptions subsequently marked as stuttering had previously been marked as normal, thus increasing Group II's Index of Confusion under instructions to mark stuttered interruptions.

The data were also analyzed to determine whether the two groups, regardless of the order of instructions, responded similarly to the eight categories of interruptions from most to fewest inconsistent responses. A rank-difference correlation coefficient was computed between the Indexes of Confusion on the eight categories of interruptions obtained for (a) Group I when instructed to mark stuttered interruptions and (b) Group II when instructed to mark stuttered interruptions. A correlation coefficient of .90 was obtained between the two sets of indexes. When instructed to mark stuttered interruptions, subjects in both groups tended to have fewest inconsistent responses on syllable repetitions and prolongations and most inconsistent responses on revisions.

A rank-difference correlation coefficient was also computed between the Indexes of Confusion on the eight types of interruptions obtained when (a) Group I was instructed to mark normal interruptions and (b) Group II was instructed to mark normal interruptions. The correlation coefficient obtained here was .85. When instructed to mark normal interruptions, subjects in both groups tended to have fewest inconsistent responses on revisions and most inconsistent responses on syllable repetitions and prolongations.

It may be concluded that the order of the eight categories when ranked from most to fewest inconsistent responses was similar for the two groups when given the *same* instructions regardless of the *order* of instructions.

Discussion

The subjects in this study demonstrated attitudes toward the different types of nonfluencies that have implications both theoretically and clinically. Some types were more often considered to be stuttering; other types were thought to be essentially normal; still other types shifted back and forth from one classification to the other, depending upon the set of the listener.

It is difficult to reconcile these findings by an examination of the characteristics of the nonfluency itself. Reasonably, there is no apparent basis for assuming that any one type of nonfluency is any more undesirable than any other one. The fact that the subjects judged certain types to be diagnostically different, that is, 'stuttered' or 'normal,' would seem to reflect an attitude of the society in which they live, rather than any basically deviant characteristic of the nonfluency.

Syllable repetitions and prolongations were more consistently identified as 'stuttering.' This fact is in agreement with other experimental findings (1, 2). Also, it has been observed clinically many times that the existence of syllable repetition in a child's speech is considered as evidence that he is a 'stutterer.' This raises an important consideration. Does a child repeat syllables, for example, *because* he is a 'stutterer,' or is he considered to be a 'stutterer' *because* he repeats syllables?

On the basis of this study, it is suggested that the cause and effect relationship may work to a degree in both directions. Apparently, he could become known as a 'stutterer' *because* he repeats syllables. Once, however, he is identified as a 'stutterer,' then his word and phrase repetitions, interjections and even revisions, to a certain extent, also come to be considered as 'stuttering,' seemingly for no other

reason than *because* he is now thought of as a 'stutterer.'[1]

Summary

When subjects were instructed to listen to a recorded speech and mark stuttered interruptions, they marked many of the same interruptions that they marked when instructed to listen to the same speech and to mark normal interruptions. They tended to 'hear' what they were instructed to listen for at the time.

The group of subjects instructed to mark stuttered interruptions first marked more interruptions as stuttered than they subsequently marked as normal. Conversely, the group instructed to mark normal interruptions first marked more as normal than they subsequently marked as stuttered.

Of the types of interruptions used in this study, subjects in both groups tended to respond most consistently, relatively speaking, to syllable repetitions, prolongations and revisions; syllable repetitions and prolongations

---

[1] One of the objectives in counseling the parents of a child who is considered to be 'stuttering' is to help them re-evaluate some of the child's speech interruptions. It has proved profitable to the present authors, at least, first to acquaint the parents with the concept of normal speech and then to ask them to pay particular attention to and to keep track of the normal interruptions in their child's speaking behavior. Often, the parents, when faced with the task of listening for and noting normal interruptions, not only become more interested in what constitutes a normal interruption, but begin classifying more of the interruptions as 'normal.' As a consequence, the number of interruptions reacted to as 'stuttering' is reduced.

167

were most consistently responded to as stuttered interruptions while revisions were most consistently responded to as normal.

Acknowledgments

The assistance of James Bost, graduate assistant, Indiana University, and of Van C. Kussrow, Instructor of Speech, Valparaiso University, in the collection of the data is gratefully acknowledged.

References

1. BOEHMLER, R. M., A quantitative study of the extensional definition of stuttering with special references to the audible designata. Ph.D. Dissertation, State University of Iowa, 1953.
2. GIOLAS, T. G. and WILLIAMS, D. E., Children's reactions to nonfluencies in adult speech. *JSHR*, 1, 1958, 86-93.
3. TUTHILL, C. E., A quantitative study of extensional meaning with special reference to stuttering. *Speech Monographs*, 13 (1), 1946, 81-98.
4. WEST, ROBERT, ANSBERRY, M., and CARR, A., *The Rehabilitation of Speech*. New York: Harper and Brothers, 1957 (3rd edition).

Evaluation and Stuttering, Part I: Speech Characteristics of Young Children

M . E . W I N G A T E

This article is the first in a series of three which undertakes a critique of the evaluational theory of stuttering (as enunciated by Johnson and others) on the basis of the very substantial amount of pertinent research that has accumulated. Although this theory has gained wide currency, there is reason to believe that a comprehensive review and reinterpretation of the research data will throw fresh light on the implications of the theory. Such review is particularly appropriate in view of the fact that the greatest proportion of the literature bearing on the issue has been presented or interpreted as favorable to the evaluational theory.

As stated by Bloodstein, Jaeger, and Tureen (1):

> Johnson's theory of stuttering will be recognized to involve essentially three assumptions:
> 1. Most normal young children speak with a considerable amount of repetition and other breaks in fluency.
> 2. Adults differ in their standards of fluency, and some react to the hesitant speech of children with unusual intolerance.
> 3. Children who are penalized for normal nonfluencies are likely to develop stuttering.

Implicit and explicit in the literature on the evaluational theory are certain extensions of these assumptions (10, 12, 13, 14, 15, 16). An extension which has been made of the first assumption is that the nonfluencies observed among children are generally similar in character and that they are thus normal. Extensions of the second assumption are: (a) that the evaluating adult makes indiscriminative use of a label, 'stuttering,' which serves to aggravate the situation, and (b) that under most circumstances this label is applied by a lay person who, being unfamiliar with or untrained in recognizing what constitutes normal fluency, uses the label incorrectly. An extension of the third assumption is that the child interiorizes this evaluation of his speech, develops anxiety and embarrassment about his (normal) nonfluencies and thus increasingly aggravates the problem.

There is a considerable amount of literature, of both a descriptive and experimental nature, which can be interpreted as providing a general basis for the credibility of the evaluation theory. To accord with the statement of assumptions as listed above, such publications may be grouped under three categories: (a) those which supply information regarding the object of 'evaluation,' namely, the speech of children; (b) those which report on the sources of 'evaluation,' i.e., the forces which bear on the developing child; and (c) those which treat spe-

M. E. Wingate (Ph.D., University of Washington, 1956) is Assistant Professor of Speech, University of Washington.

JOURNAL OF SPEECH AND HEARING DISORDERS, 1962, Vol. 27, pp. 106-115.

cifically the issue of nonfluency and the effect of evaluation of nonfluency. There is some amount of overlap among the studies pertinent to each of these three categories, particularly in regard to the latter two, but for the purposes of organization, the material will be presented in three sections.

In this first section, inquiry will be addressed to studies under the first category, those which center around the first stated assumption of the evaluation theory and the corollary it contains.

Nonfluencies in Children

There is no little amount of material in the literature which can be interpreted as supporting the premise that most young children show 'repetition or other nonfluency' in their speech. The reports by Fisher (7), Metraux (17), Davis (4, 5), Branscom et al. (3), Oxtoby (18), Johnson (10, 13, 14, 16), Steer (20), and Egland (6), have frequently been cited as substantiating this point. A careful analysis of these reports, however, reveals that while their findings do permit the generalization that nonfluencies of some kind occur among many young children, they certainly do not support the extensions of this generalization which, unfortunately, are frequently inferred and implied.

These extensions are essentially of two kinds: (a) that nonfluencies are *common* among youngsters, i.e., not only that most children evidence nonfluencies but also that the frequency of occurrence is generally comparable among children; and (b) that the nonfluencies are generally similar in character from one child to another. In fact, such generalizations have become common coin, casually spent, as reflected in the following randomly selected instances. Sheehan, in an article (19) bearing on an entirely different aspect of stuttering research refers to '. . . the stage of hesitancy and syllable repetition through which nearly all children seem to pass.' Sheehan's statement appears to identify syllable repetitions and hesitations as the common nonfluencies. Johnson in *The Onset of Stuttering* (16, p. 144) says,

> . . . the control group parents who did report nonfluencies were evidently referring to the ordinary repetitions and hesitations generally characteristic in varying measure of the speech of young children, and so of the speech of the rest of the control group children, too.

This statement employs the general term 'repetitions,' but further, it says that even though some of the control group children were *not* reported by their parents to have shown 'repetitions,' these children must nevertheless have shown 'repetitions' since this is characteristic of young children. Statements of this kind, equally unwarranted and unsupported, are multiplied throughout the literature as well as in casual professional exchange and in professional training situations.

Referring to irregularities in children's speech with a general term such an 'nonfluencies' or 'repetitions' may be a verbal convenience, as well as a theoretical fortuity, but it obscures some very important facts about the nature of speech irregularities. The practice of referring broadly to 'repetitions' implicitly dismisses the potentially very significant observation that repetitions differ in kind (sound, syllable, word, or phrase repetitions) and in amount (number of repetitions per instance of occurrence, as well as overall frequency of repetition). The significance of these differences should be manifest following a review of the above-mentioned literature. Such review is indicated to demonstrate that contrary to common practice, strict qualifications are demanded in any reference to the findings of these studies, in that most of them contain more than a suggestion that differences in 'repetitions' do exist and have great potential significance.

Speech Characteristics of Normal-speaking Children. Fisher (7) studied the language and speech characteristics of 72 children between the ages of two and five years. References in the literature which cite Fisher's report as supporting the normality of 'repetitions' undoubtedly refer to her statement that repetitions of speech patterns are characteristic of very young children and that these repetitions in the speech of preschool children tend to decrease with age. However, it is highly questionable to what extent her remarks can be accepted as bearing specifically on the issue. First, she defined repetition as '. . . exact repetition of the same remark, verbal or nonverbal, with no variation in word or sound pattern.' She also speaks of the children as 'continuing to experiment with repetitions,' relating this to children's reported interest in having things (sayings, stories) repeated to them, as well as to their apparent enjoyment of intentionally repeating nonsense words, sound patterns, new words, humorous remarks, and the like. Thus 'repetitions' at least include intentional repeating of larger verbal groupings in the manner of play. At the same time, she reported finding marked individual differences in 'repeti-tions' and more frequent repetitions in boys than in girls.

Metraux (*17*), in a source less frequently cited than others, described the speech characteristics of 207 young children on several dimensions, including 'repetitions.' She reported that 18-month-old children repeat syllables or words more often than not. At 24 months there is occasional syllable repetition and use of 'a' before many remarks, but the most common characteristic is repetition of a word or phrase, sometimes with variation; there is much variation from child to child. At 30 months most children repeat a word or phrase occasionally; *some* continue 'interminably' with increased force, pitch, and volume. The focus here appeared to be in the child's attempt to make personal-social contact and relates to the child's interest in repetition and his demand for repetition from others. Some children evidence 'developmental stuttering' at this age, with first-word or syllable repetitions which frequently progress to a mild tonic block that is easily broken.

According to Metraux, at 30 months most children are 'on an easy repetitive basis,' with only occasional repetition of a beginning syllable and some instances of word repetition within a sentence; tonic blocking is infrequent. Repetitions (type unspecified) were reported to be most frequent at 42 months and to have the 'somewhat compulsive quality' noted at 30 months. The repetition at 42 months often seems to be in relation to another person in demand for attention, information, or encouragement. General rate of speech seems to be faster in this period, and 'developmental stuttering' is again prominent, with breathing sometimes

171

noticeably disturbed. But, '. . . more individual variations begin to appear with children whose tensional overflow affects the speech.' At 48 months children show little repetition except for an occasional phrase. At the same time, 'The child whose speech has been characterized by periods of developmental stuttering up to this time, however, may continue to have phases when repetition and blocking occur.' At 54 months children often interject at the beginning of a phrase but seldom repeat except for emphasis. However, the child who evidenced speech blocking earlier may still have occasional difficulty.

Metraux's article is not sufficiently explicit regarding the types of repetition observed, but it is certainly adequate to demonstrate that (a) all, or even most, children do not show the same kinds of repetition nor with comparable frequency, (b) that syllable repetitions are not common, and (c) that certain children exhibit more extremes in nonfluency which persist over relatively long periods of time.

Davis (4, 5), studying 62 nonstuttering preschoolers, age two to five, concluded that 'repetition' is a part of the speech pattern of all children; but she also reported her data as revealing that the amount and kind of repetition differed from child to child. She found, further, that although repetition of words and phrases decreased with age, syllable repetitions were not affected by age. In addition, at all ages, syllable repetitions occurred much less frequently than either word or phrase repetitions (a ratio of 1:3:6). At the same time, the number of repetitions per instance of occurrence for syllable repetitions was more than twice as great as for word repetitions and more than three times as great as for phrase repetitions. Almost half of the children studied showed no syllable repetition of two or more in extent; yet in contrast to this Davis found that syllable repetitions stood out as the type in which more than half of the instances of repetition fell 'in what might be termed the "extreme extent range." ' She also found more instances of syllable repetitions in boys. The following quotations from Davis (4) are relevant in regard to the kind of repetitions which might be considered normal:

This material would tend to show that a child whose speech is such that approximately one word in four is a repeated word, either in part or in whole in a word or phrase repetition, is not presenting any abnormality in speech, but is talking 'normally.'

In consideration of the instances of syllable repetition in terms of verbal output a very different picture was presented.

In consideration of all these measures it was found that the two which deal with the instances of syllable repetition and with the number of repetitive syllables used in syllable repetitions, were the best measures for determining the children who deviated markedly from the group. In each of these measures the child who was termed a 'stutterer' stands out dramatically from the balance of the group.

Branscom et al. (3) summarized the findings of four studies on nonfluency in 193 nonstuttering preschool children (ages two to six). This report included the studies of Davis and Oxtoby. In a summary of the frequency of syllable, word, and phrase repetitions recorded in three of the studies which appraised speech behavior in a free-play situation, the values provide a ratio of approximately 1:2:3; that is, syllable repetitions occurred less than half as

172

often as word repetitions and less than a third as often as phrase repetitions. This report mentioned also that word repetition correlated to some extent with both syllable repetition and phrase repetition but that nonsignificant correlation between syllable repetition and phrase repetition indicated a lack of relationship between these two types. In Oxtoby's study, statistical comparison was made between boys and girls on four repetition measures (syllable, word, phrase, and total), among which only one difference approached significance at the 10 per cent level of confidence—boys showed more syllable repetitions than girls.

Comparisons of Young Stutterers and Nonstutterers. In his earlier study comparing stuttering and nonstuttering children, Johnson (*10*) obtained information on 46 stutterers between the approximate ages of two and nine years and a like group of nonstutterers. His report dealt mainly with history and developmental data from which he stated that the two groups were essentially similar.[1] He did not present any detailed data on the speech characteristics of the two groups, but in a summary statement of this aspect he said,

> . . . it is sufficient to say that in approximately 92 per cent of the [stuttering] cases the first phenomena that were diagnosed as stuttering were beyond doubt essentially effortless repetitions of words, phrases, or the first sounds or syllables of words. In other cases also, these phenomena were, so far as could be determined, the predominating features, although there is some question as to whether, in these cases, diagnoses of stuttering were made before the child had begun to exhibit some degree of hypertonicity in con-

nection with the repetitions or before the child had begun to exhibit such other reactions as prolongations of sounds, conspicuous pauses, etc.

Thus, at least prolongations and conspicuous pauses were evidently features distinguishing the stutterers from nonstutterers.[2]

Steer (*20*), in a comparison of a group of 30 preschool stutterers (ages three to six) with a group of 20 like-age normal speaking children, described a number of symptoms of breathing disturbance observed in both groups. Although concluding that both stutterers and nonstutterers evidenced disturbances in breathing while speaking, his analysis revealed a different type of breathing irregularity for the stutterers than for the nonstutterers.

Egland (*6*) evaluated the occurrence of nonfluencies in a group of 26 non-stuttering kindergarten children to which he compared similar observations from three preschool age stutterers. Somewhat contrary to results mentioned earlier, he reported for his non-stuttering group a higher frequency of sound or syllable repetitions than either word or phrase repetitions and no marked differences between boys and girls as to type of repetition. Repetitions of parts of words constituted the most common type of repetitious speech in both stutterers and nonstutterers. However, the stutterers showed a markedly higher percentage of repetitions of all types; their repetitions consisted more heavily of sound or syllable repetitions and very few phrase repetitions; and they showed more repetition units per instance of repetition. Also,

---

[1]Except that there were more stutterers in the families of the stutterers.

[2]Details from this study are included in a more recent publication by Johnson (*16*), which is reviewed later in this article.

the speech samples of the nonstutterers contained a higher percentage of 'stalls' ('ah,' 'um,' etc.) whereas the speech of the stutterers had a greater percentage of prolongations.

In Johnson's major work on this issue (16), he reports on three separate studies which drew comparisons between nonstuttering children and children 'regarded as stutterers.' The combined samples contained 246 children in each group, over an age range of approximately two to 14 years. The findings of differences in speech characteristics reveal that the experimental ('regarded as stutterers') group evidenced significantly more syllable repetitions, whereas the control group showed significantly more phrase repetitions. Further, significantly more experimental children evidenced prolongations whereas significantly more control group children showed nonfluencies of the order of silent intervals, pauses, or interjections. Although Johnson stresses and elaborates on the overlap between the two groups on the various kinds of nonfluencies, the fact that all of the above differences were significant at the one per cent level seems the more noteworthy findings; this is particularly true in view of the above studies which indicate that it is essentially in terms of sound and syllable repetitions and prolongations that stutterers differ from nonstutterers.

Johnson's most recent report on a study of this type (11) deals with adults, but it is included in the present discussion because of the relevance of its content. Johnson obtained comparisons between 100 stuttering and 100 nonstuttering college age adults (50 males and 50 females in each group) on a number of measures of 'disfluency.' It is pertinent to note initially that special statistics were employed in treating the data because of the considerable skew in the distributions. This fact in itself provides a commentary on the 'normality' of disfluencies, particularly certain kinds. Even so, nonstutterers were in general 'considerably less disfluent than the stutterers.' Again, the results revealed the stutterers to evidence very many more 'part word repetitions' (sound and syllable repetitions) than the nonstutterers.

Concerning prolongations, Johnson (11, pp. 7-8) expressed the comparison inversely and in terms of proportions:

> The proportions of both major groups presenting no broken words or prolonged sounds were sufficiently large to warrant the statement that approximately half of the stutterers were indistinguishable from most of the nonstutterers with respect to these types of disfluency.

Even when expressed in this manner it seems clear that prolongations were much more characteristic of the stutterers. Further, his tabled data reveal that, as an average for the three conditions of the study, the stuttering group showed 43.7 prolongations per 100 words, whereas the nonstuttering group showed only 3.6 prolongations per 100 words.

Johnson reported 'virtually complete' overlap between the two groups in respect to revisions. He reported 'considerably extensive' overlap for interjections, incomplete phrases, and word and phrase repetitions. On all of the latter four measures, stutterers exceeded nonstutterers, but only slightly on word repetitions and very little on phrase repetitions and incomplete phrases.[3] Stutterers were recorded as evidencing considerably more interjections, but this finding requires qualification: interjections differ quite a bit in quality—a single 'uh,' for example, is not uncommonly used by normal speakers as a pause-filler while searching for the right word, whereas 'uh uh uh' has the definite quality of a sound repetition. Interjections also differ in terms of the amount of effort or struggle involved. In Johnson's tabulation, an 'uh' or an 'uh uh uh' were each counted as one instance of interjection, and no notation was made regarding associated effort.

All of the differences found in this study would be enhanced, of course, by taking into account the substantial difference between the two groups on amount of verbal output (the stutterers showed markedly lower verbal output than the nonstutterers).

Voelker (21) studied the speech fluency of 62 nonstuttering orphanage adolescents age 12 to 19 and compared their speech characteristics with those of seven stutterers of similar age. He reported a wide range of fluency in his normal group, with some individuals showing some kind of 'break' every 2.3 words and others having a 'break' only once in every 12.5 words. He found a sex difference, with girls showing 20 per cent fewer breaks and having smoother speech, the boys being more subject to hesitation and repeti-

[3]It seems meaningless to point out that stutterers are not easily distinguished from nonstutterers in respect to these irregularities. This only serves to indicate that stutterers also show 'normal' nonfluencies. The important point remains that there is a very remarkable difference between stutterers and nonstutterers in respect to sound and syllable repetitions and prolongations.

tion. However, he found that the average speaker had no syllable repetitions per 100 words and less than one word or phrase repetition per 100 words. They also had very few other kinds of 'breaks,' although hesitations (10 per 100 words) and conspicuous pauses (three to six per 100 words) were relatively prominent. The stutterers, on the other hand, showed a fluency break every 1.2 words to every 3.7 words; compared to the normals, the mean fluency rating was in the lowest decile, with their scores on half of the measures of nonfluency being subnormal. The stutterers were not equally nonfluent in all aspects of fluency; e.g., they were actually slightly above the average in number of conspicuous pauses, and they did not have notably more hesitations. However, on syllable and word repetitions and prolongations they were definitely abnormal. Voelker (21) commented that fluency is a broader term than stuttering, and that while it is evident that stutterers have a defect in fluency, lowness in fluency per se does not necessarily mean stuttering. He predicted that as research continues to add to our knowledge of stuttering, it will ultimately be realized that '. . . when stuttering is defined as a defect of fluency, defects in prolongations, syllable repetitions, and word repetitions are the referends.'

The analysis of the foregoing studies of the speech characteristics of children thus reveals that among those children who evidence fluency irregularities there is considerable variation both in amount and in type. Further, some of these children exhibit much more of the kinds of 'nonfluency' seen most often in individuals acknowledged to be stutterers. These findings are consistent with the results of a study by Glasner and Vermilyea (9), who investigated how the term 'primary stuttering' was defined and employed by 171 professional workers in the field of speech pathology. In their replies these workers revealed variation and uncertainty in their definition and use of the term, due largely to the complication presented by their effort to give consideration to the factors of awareness, struggle, and secondary mannerisms. However, the over-all results of the study indicated that regardless of whether or not, or how, the term was used '. . . a substantial [87] per cent of the workers who replied feel that there is definitely something in the speech of some young children that compels both parents *and* therapists to do *something* about it.'

From the studies reviewed above, it would appear that the 'something in the speech of some young children' mentioned by Glasner and Vermilyea consists predominantly of syllable repetitions and prolongations.[4] This interpretation is supported by several other studies which bear on the issue from a different direction. These studies indicate, consistent with Voelker's prediction, that syllable repetitions and prolongations are the referents when the term *stuttering* is employed. For instance, Boehmler (2) reported that both trained and untrained judges labeled sound and syllable repetitions as stuttering more often than they did revisions and interjections, regardless

of the rated severity of nonfluency of the speech samples judged. Williams and Kent (22) found that their untrained judges shifted their judgments of speech interruptions somewhat according to whether they were given a set to judge speech samples as containing 'normal' interruptions or 'stuttered' interruptions. Even so, they most consistently judged syllable repetitions and prolongations as 'stuttered' and revisions as 'normal.'

Giolas and Williams (8) have demonstrated that even young children show similar reactions. Kindergarten and second grade children listened to stories recorded with a Fluent Pattern, an Interjections Pattern, and a Repetitions Pattern. The kindergarten children were less consistent than the second graders in choosing between the two nonfluent patterns, but they preferred the fluent pattern. The second graders placed the Fluent Pattern first, the Interjections Pattern second, and the Repetitions Pattern last in order of desirability. They were more specific in indicating dislike for speech interruptions, particularly repetitions, and they more often used the term 'stuttering' in referring to the Repetitions Pattern.

Summary

This article reviews the research which has previously been cited as partial substantiation of the evaluational theory of stuttering. It finds a consistent basis for interpreting the findings of this research as actually contradictory to the first assumption of the evaluational theory. Specifically, the pertinent research data is seen as refuting the claims and implications, fundamental to the evaluational theory,

---

[4]Glasner and Vermilyea's data support this deduction, in that 36 per cent of their respondents mentioned these characteristics specifically, another 20 per cent did not distinguish between primary and secondary stuttering, and another 11 per cent viewed primary stuttering as 'a stage of stuttering.'

that fluency irregularities are common to nearly all children, and the derived contentions (a) that children are generally similar in the extent and kind of nonfluency they evidence, and (b) that these 'normal nonfluencies' are generally no different from those observed in individuals 'identified as stutterers.'

First, it seems evident that children do show considerable individual variation in the type, amount, and frequency of their fluency irregularities. Second, certain kinds of fluency irregularities are found much more frequently in children 'identified as stutterers' and also are quite consistently identified as not normal, whereas other kinds of fluency irregularities are characteristic of nonstutterers and also are quite consistently identified as normal.

These findings demand recognition of the fact that it is misleading as well as confusing to lump all kinds of fluency irregularities under a general referent, such as 'nonfluency' or 'repetitions and other nonfluencies,' and that this practice obscures important differences among children which can be and have been demonstrated.

In presenting the available evidence as contradictory to the contention of the commonness and similarity of fluency irregularities in children, this analysis indicates to the author that the first assumption of the evaluational theory of stuttering is untenable. Implications of this analysis relevant to other pertinent areas of research and to the over-all issue of evaluation and stuttering will be developed in a subsequent paper.

References

1. BLOODSTEIN, O., JAEGER, W., and TUREEN, J., A study of the diagnosis of stuttering by parents of stutterers and non-stutterers. *J. Speech Hearing Dis.*, 17, 1952, 308-316.

2. BOEHMLER, R. M., Listener responses to non-fluencies. *J. Speech Hearing Res.*, 1, 1958, 132-141.

3. BRANSCOM, MARGARET E., HUGHES, JEANNETTE, and OXTOBY, E. T., Studies of nonfluency in the speech of preschool children. In W. Johnson, (Ed.) *Stuttering in Children and Adults*. Minneapolis, Minn.: University of Minnesota Press, 1955.

4. DAVIS, D. M., The relation of repetitions in the speech of young children to certain measures of language maturity and situational factors: Part I. *J. Speech Dis.*, 4, 1939, 303-318.

5. DAVIS, D. M., The relation of repetitions in the speech of young children to certain measures of language maturity and situational factors: Part II and Part III. *J. Speech Dis.*, 5, 1940, 235-246.

6. EGLAND, G. O., Repetitions and prolongations in the speech of stuttering and nonstuttering children. In W. Johnson (Ed.), *Stuttering in Children and Adults*. Minneapolis, Minn.: University of Minnesota Press, 1955.

7. FISHER, MARY S., Language patterns of pre-school children. *J. Exp. Education*, 1, 1932, 70-86.

8. GIOLAS, T. G., and WILLIAMS, D. E., Children's reactions to nonfluencies in adult speech. *J. Speech Hearing Res.*, 1, 1958, 86-93.

9. GLASNER, P. J., and VERMILYEA, FRANA D., An investigation of the definition and use of the diagnosis, 'primary stuttering.' *J. Speech Hearing Dis.*, 18, 1953, 161-168.

10. JOHNSON, W., A study of the onset and development of stuttering. *J. Speech Dis.*, 7, 1942, 251-257.

11. JOHNSON, W., Measurements of oral reading and speaking rate and disfluency of adult male and female stutterers and nonstutterers. *J. Speech Hearing Dis.*, Monograph Supplement 7, 1961.

12. JOHNSON, W., *People In Quandaries: The Semantics of Personal Adjustment*, New York: Harper, 1946.

13. JOHNSON, W., (Ed.), *Stuttering in Children and Adults*. Minneapolis, Minn.: University of Minnesota Press, 1955.

14. JOHNSON, W., The Indians have no word for it: I. Stuttering in children. *Quart. J. Speech.*, 30, 1944, 330-337.

15. JOHNSON, W., et al., *Speech Handicapped School Children*, New York: Harper, 1956.

16. JOHNSON, W., et al., *The Onset of Stuttering*. Minneapolis, Minn.: University of Minnesota Press, 1959.

17. METRAUX, RUTH W., Speech profiles of the pre-school child 18 to 54 months. *J. Speech Hearing Dis.*, 15, 1950, 37-53.

18. OXTOBY, E. T., A quantitative study of repetition in the speech of three-year-old children. Unpublished M.A. Thesis, Univ. Iowa, 1943.

19. SHEEHAN, J. G., Projective studies of stuttering. *J. Speech Hearing Dis.*, 23, 1958, 18-25.

20. STEER, M. D., Symptomatologies of young stutterers. *J. Speech Dis.*, 2, 1937, 3-13.

21. VOELKER, C. H., A preliminary investigation for a normative study of fluency, a clinical index to the severity of stuttering. *Am. J. Orthopsy.*, 14, 1944, 285-294.

22. WILLIAMS, D. E., and KENT, LOUISE R., Listener evaluations of speech interruptions. *J. Speech Hearing Res.*, 1, 1958, 124-131.

SPEAKING FLUENCY IN THE PARENTS
OF STUTTERERS AND NON-STUTTERERS

Kenneth J. Knepflar, Ph.D.

Interest in this study was first stimulated when I observed what seemed to be an unusual amount of speaking disfluency among a number of parents of stutterers during intake interviews and parent conferences. Statements like: "Well, no, uh, there hasn't there hasn't been any stuttering in our, in our, in our family!" made me begin searching the literature in an attempt to find reports of clinical observations or research studies that would relate to my own observations. No relevant research evidence was uncovered and only a few brief statements were found of clinical observations similar to my own. Bloodstein, for example, made this observation:

> "Occasionally, parents who asserted that there
> was no stuttering in the family, had so many
> pauses, repetitions and other breaks in fluency
> in their own speech that they aroused the sus-
> picion that they had not been entirely candid."

While prior to this study there has been no experimental evidence concerning disfluency in parents of stutterers, per se, a number of past research findings that relate to my study should be mentioned briefly.

Davis and Egland have both demonstrated the existence of disfluencies of various kinds during the normal development of speech and language.

Wingate and Van Riper have both pointed out that these disfluencies may be different in kind and degree in children who tend to be identified as stutterers.

Johnson and his associates have shown the existence of disfluencies in the speech of adult non-stutterers.

Since these disfluent, normal-speaking adults provide both the biological hereditary make-up and the speech environments for their children, it would seem of vital importance that we know if there are any differences with regard to disfluency of those adults who produce stutterers and those who have children with no speech problems.

My study, then, is based on the fundamental question. "Do the parents of stutterers differ in speaking fluency from the parents of non-stutterers?"

ADAPTED FROM A PAPER PRESENTED AT THE 41ST ANNUAL CONVENTION AMERICAN SPEECH AND HEARING ASSOCIATION, Chicago Ill., 31,1965.

Twenty-one mothers and twenty-one fathers of stutterers
were matched according to ages, educational levels and numbers
of children per family with twenty-one mothers and twenty-one
fathers of children who have never stuttered or exhibited any
kind of speech problem. Samples of conversational speech, based
on a selection by each subject from a list of ten speaking topics,
were tape recorded individually. Family history information was
acquired by means of structured interviews following the recording
sessions.

All eighty-four recordings were judged independently by two
speech-therapist judges according to the eight types of disfluency listed by Johnson and his associates in their 1961 Journal
of Speech and Hearing Disorders supplement report. These eight
types were: interjections of sounds, syllables, words, and phrases
such as uh, er, well and mm, part-word repetitions, word repetitions,
phrase repetitions, revisions, incomplete phrases, broken words,
and prolonged sounds. Because of the infrequency of occurrence
of some disfluency types, two types were eliminated and others
were grouped together, so that, for purposes of statistical analysis, three types of disfluency were used. These were: interjections, repetitions, and revisions.

A Pearson product-moment correlation coefficient was computed between the two judges' scores based on 200 word speech
samples from all 84 subjects. The disfluency data were subjected
to an analysis of variance (Lindquist Type VI Design) in which
the three variables were:

1. Groups--parents of stutterers vs. parents of
    normal speakers.
2. Types of disfluency.
3. Sex--mothers vs. fathers.

There was a high correlation between the scores of the two
judges. For interjections, .943; for repetitions, .914; and for
revisions, .741.

The analysis of variance showed the following results:

1. The parents of stutterers display more disflu-
    encies than the parents of non-stutters (sig-
    nificant at the .025 level).
2. Interjections occur with greater frequency in all
    subsamples than repetitions and revisions (signifi-
    cant at the .001 level).
3. Fathers produce approximately the same number of
    disfluencies in their speech as mothers.
4. Fathers of stutterers differ from fathers of non-
    stutterers in the same amount and direction as
    mothers of stutterers differ from the mothers of
    non-stutterers.

180

5. The relative incidence of different types of disfluencies is not the same for mothers as for fathers, in that the excess of interjections is greater for fathers than for mothers (significant at the .01 level).
6. More interjections, as compared to the other types of disfluency, occur among the parents of stutterers than among the parents of non-stutterers (significant at the .01 level).
7. Fathers of stutterers show substantially more interjections than any other subsample and the mothers of stutterers produce more revisions. The four subsamples exhibited similar numbers of repetitions (significant at the .025 level).

On the basis of these results, the fundamental question, upon which this research is based, must be answered affirmatively: the parents of stutterers do differ in speaking fluency from the parents of non-stutterers.

Before discussing some of the implications of my research, I would like to present an interesting side-light of the study. An analysis of the post-recording interview results revealed that six of the fathers of stutterers reported that they currently stuttered, or had stuttered in the past. If these six individuals were to be included in the experimental group sample, it seemed important to compare the disfluency data for them with the findings for the entire subgroup to which they belonged. This comparison demonstrated that the disfluency means for the six stuttering fathers were only 2/3 as great as those for the entire experimental sub-group of fathers of stutterers. The reported diffferences between parents of stutterers and non-stutterers cannot be explained, therefore, in terms of the inclusion of parents who stutter in the experimental group. On the contrary, this suggests the possibility that while stutterers may have disfluencies that are different in kind from non-stutterers, they may often have fewer total interruptions in the smooth flow of speech.

Since the completion of this study, another interesting observation has been made. Speech samples of several stutterers have been analyzed as to number of disfluencies. These disfluency data have been compared to those of both parents of each stutterer. In several instances, one or both parents had a greater number of disfluencies per 100 words than did their child who stutters.

It is apparent that these research findings have theoretical implications for those who explain the high familial incidence of stuttering on the basis of familial diathesis and those who explain it on the basis of cultural factors. Time today limits discussion of these etiological implications, but I shall mention a few practical implications that have specific meaning for all of us, regardless of theoretical bias.

First, speech clinicians should be aware of the kinds of speech stimulation a child is receiving at home. If, for example, parents are expecting unrealistically high speech fluency standards from their children, it would seem possible that training them to recognize and accept their own disfluencies as normal phenomena, would aid in helping them to accept the presence of disfluencies in the speech of their child. In many instances, parents have been shown how to produce easy, comfortable voluntary disfluencies in their speech, so that the child's speech environment is conducive to the production of normally disfluent speech.

Older stutterers have actually been taught to recognize the various types of disfluencies in speech samples of their own parents. In most instances, this is an eye-opening experience, since stutterers usually seem to be impressed with the adequacy of the speech of their parents.

Stutterers have also been taught to produce voluntary normal disfluencies on non-feared words, thus lowering their fluency standards. In many cases, stutterers have identified all of their own disfluencies as moments of stuttering, even those which are perfectly comfortable, with no evidence of struggle or avoidance.

I also suggest that we, as speech therapists, are often not aware of the frequency of disfluencies in our own speech. An ability to handle disfluencies well in his own speech, and to produce them voluntarily, can make the clinician a much more appropriate speech model for stutterers.

It is hoped that additional related studies, and perhaps a replication of this study, will be conducted so that these findings can be either supported, or negated. Until that time, I, for one, am grateful for the opportunity of having some additional research information, which has had a direct bearing on my clinical handling of both stutterers and their parents.

<u>Voluntary Normal Disfluency: A Speech</u>
<u>Therapy Technique For Stutterers</u>

Adapted From a Paper Presented For the 41st Annual Convention,
American Speech and Hearing Association
Chicago, Illinois, October 31, 1965.

Kenneth J. Knepflar, Ph. D.

A number of techniques have been recommended as symptom modification approaches to stuttering. One of the most frequently quoted is
the concept of voluntary stuttering, originally described by Knight
Dunlap as an application of his negative practice concept. He suggested
that stutterers study their specific types of involuntary spasms, copy
them as nearly as possible, and then stutter voluntarily.

The earlier writings of Van Riper, Johnson, Bryngelson and Travis
also recommended the use of various types of voluntary stuttering.
Most of these approaches involved variations of an easy bouncing or
prolongation of sounds on non-feared words. Some recommend them
as methods of handling stuttered words, or replacing old stuttering
patterns with new more acceptable approaches to stuttered words.

Variations of the voluntary stuttering concept are still included
in the therapeutic frameworks of many clinicians who deal with those
who stutter. It has been the experience of many clinicians, myself
included, that voluntary stuttering can be a beneficial technique when
used appropriately in a well integrated program of therapy for certain stutterers. Unfortunately, however, voluntary stuttering carries

with it a number of therapeutic risks and clinical pitfalls which may be frustrating to both the stutterer and his therapist. These negative features include:

1. The possible use of voluntary stuttering as a crutch, which achieves only temporary relief, if not skillfully directed by therapists.

2. The failure of stutterers to use voluntary stuttering at times when it is most needed - in difficult feared speaking situations.

3. The emotional resistance, which the introduction of voluntary stuttering frequently involves, when stutterers are asked to exhibit purposely their most feared and most hated problem.

The therapeutic technique presented in this paper is not to be thought of as an adaptation of voluntary stuttering, either by clinicians or by stutterers. This technique, voluntary normal disfluency, is based upon recent research findings and upon factors concerning normal speech which have been known, but heretofore largely ignored in reported therapeutic approaches to the stuttering problem.

Davis, Egland, and others have demonstrated that children display disfluencies of various kinds during the normal development

of speech and language. Disfluencies have also been shown by Johnson
and others to exist in the speech of normally speaking adults. Both
Van Riper and Wingate report that the disfluencies that occur normally
in children are different in kind and degree from those that occur in
children who stutter.

My own recent research, A Study of Speaking Fluency in the Parents
of Stutterers and Non-Stutterers, has demonstrated that the parents of
stutterers exhibit more speaking disfluencies than the parents of non-
stutterers. In this research, the mean number of disfluencies of six
fathers of stutterers, who were or had been stutterers themselves, was
only 2/3 as great as the mean number of disfluencies of the entire group
of fathers of stutterers.

Speech samples of several stutterers suggest that many of them
have fewer disfluencies, although of different kinds, than either of
their normally speaking parents, yet the child has a speech problem,
the parents do not.

Stutterers, when asked to evaluate the speech of their parents or
of other individuals with excessive effortless normal disfluency, almost uniformly judge the speech as desirable and completely acceptable.

Some stutterers have expressed a belief that any interruption in the
smooth flow of their own speech is abnormal, and therefore, is responded to as stuttering.

These research findings and clinical observations have led to the development of voluntary normal disfluency as a speech therapy technique with secondary stutterers of all ages. The technique is based, in part, on the belief that abnormal disfluencies can be replaced, to some extent, at least, by normal disfluencies.

Voluntary normal disfluency is based on the assumption that all speakers possess a certain capacity for speaking fluently, based upon a number of constitutional, cultural and psychological factors, such as intelligence, expressive language ability, motor coordination, educational level, aspiration level, and frustration tolerance. It is suggested that one factor in the development of stuttering is the individual's attempt to speak beyond his particular capacity for fluency. It is believed that voluntary normal disfluency is one technique which can lower the stutterer's fluency standards, which are often unrealistically high, and thus aid him in tolerating the existence of disfluencies in his speech pattern.

Introduction of the technique should always be preceded by some ear training, so that stutterers become aware of the existence of disfluencies, particularly word and phrase repetitions, in speech samples that they judge to be normal. Recorded samples of the speech of their parents often serves this purpose. Listening for normal disfluencies in the speech of the therapist is also helpful.

Introduction of the technique should always be preceded by some ear training, so that stutterers become aware of the existence of disfluencies, particularly word and phrase repetitions, in speech samples that they judge to be normal. Recorded samples of the speech of their parents often serves this purpose. Listening for normal disfluencies in the speech of the therapist is also helpful.

The technique is always used on non-feared words upon which there is no stuttering or anticipation of stuttering.

Although there are many kinds of normal disfluency, word and phrase repetitions have been used most successfully during the initial stages. Part-word repetitions are identified by most stutterers as stuttering symptoms and, therefore, cannot be handled comfortably as voluntary normal disfluencies. Part-word repetitions and prolongations of sounds, when done purposely, must be considered voluntary stuttering, not voluntary normal disfluency.

It is believed that it is important for stutterers to accept the fact that word and phrase repetitions are perfectly acceptable characteristics in normal speech production. They are trained to recognize the differences between the easy, normal word and phrase repetitions in the flow of normal connected speech, and their abnormal usage when they are used by stutterers as postponement devices preceding a moment of stuttering.

In order to assist stutterers in monitoring their own speech and in becoming aware of the frequency of various types of voluntary normal disfluency, a tallying system has been used successfully. When this is done the stutterer is trained to tally each voluntary disfluency in one of three columns, labeled part-word repetitions, word repetitions and phrase repetitions. When part word repetitions predominate, the stutterer is instructed to attempt to increase the frequency of word and phrase repetitions, thus changing the pattern from one that is identified as stuttering to one in which normal disfluencies predominate.

Several positive effects of the use of voluntary normal disfluency, have been demonstrated:

1. Improved tolerance of moments of stuttering when they occur.

2. Increased numbers of spontaneous normal disfluencies of all kinds.

3. Gradually decreasing severity and frequency of occurrence of actual moments of stuttering.

4. Improved acceptance by stutterers of themselves as disfluent individuals with decreased fear and avoidance.

In conclusion, it is suggested that the use of voluntary normal disfluency is not presented here as a technique to be used by itself. It is presented, rather, as one technique that has been found useful as one of many clinical methods in group and individual therapy programs for stutterers, embodying both speech therapy and psychotherapeutic approaches to the problem of secondary stuttering in children and adults. Voluntary normal disfluency should not present a conflict to clinicians, regardless of theoretical bias or therapeutic approach. It requires no symptom modification. Voluntary normal disfluency is based on the belief that the disfluent characteristics of normal speech should be considered by all clinicians who work with those who stutter.

REFINEMENTS IN THE USE OF VOLUNTARY NORMAL DISFLUENCY: A FOLLOW-UP REPORT

Adapted From a Paper Presented For the 44th Annual Convention,
American Speech and Hearing Association
Denver, Colorado, November 17, 1968

Kenneth J. Knepflar, Ph. D.   Private Practice
Pasadena, California

During the past five years voluntary normal disfluency has been utilized by me with 128 stutterers, ranging from age three to fifty-nine. It has been used in conjunction with a number of other individual and group therapeutic approaches, planned to meet the varying needs of these stutterers.

The technique was first presented at the 1965 ASHA Convention and has been discussed and demonstrated since that time throughout the State of California and has been used by a number of clinicians in the public schools and in a variety of clinical settings.

Many of us have worked with those who stutter for a number of years. Few of us are completely satisfied with our clinical approaches and therapeutic results. Is it possible that we frequently overlook some very basic known factors when we diagnose and treat stutterers? Is it possible that speech pathologists, in their attempts to solve the many problems concerning stutterers, are making the problem more complex than it really is?

Is it possible that the fears and insecurities of clinicians regarding their backgrounds, training and experience in the area of stuttering is felt by the stutterer and is the major factor limiting his therapeutic progress?

Why is stuttering still referred to as a mystery, a riddle, a puzzle and an enigma, even after the publication of more than 2000 articles on the subject? If we cannot explain the problem adequately to stutterers, how can they be expected to accept it and deal with it? No one disagrees that it is desirable for stutterers to understand themselves. We must make certain that they understand their stuttering!

I believe that it may be very easy to explain why much of our research on stuttering has not shown significant differences between stutterers and non-stutterers. The reason is obvious: there <u>may be</u> <u>no significant differences between stutterers and non-stutterers</u>, at least not in the ways in which we have been searching. The difference may be that stutterers stutter: non-stutterers do not. If stuttering is a symptom of any number of disorders, then we must expect stutterers as well as non-stutterers, to run the full gamut in terms of organic factors, emotional differences and learning capacities.

If the only consistent difference between stutterers and non-stutterers is their stuttering, it would seem sensible to assume that perhaps the symptom of stuttering itself, is deserving of more attention. The main way in which stuttered speech is different from non-stuttered speech is the way in which it is disfluent. It would be easier if we could say that normal speech is fluent and that stuttered speech is disfluent..but this is not the case.

On the other hand, a number of studies have shown that normal speech may be quite disfluent. Johnson has pointed out, for example,

that some stutterers have fewer disfluencies than some non-stutterers.
My own studies are bearing this out...even to the extent that some
stutterers have fewer disfluencies per one hundred words than either
of their parents, yet the stutterer has a problem, the parents do not.
My research has demonstrated that the parents of stutterers have significantly more disluency in their speech than the parents of non-stutterers. It also demonstrated that those fathers of stutterers who
stuttered themselves, had only 2/3 as many disfluencies as those who
never stuttered.

Most of the disfluencies, which occur in normal speech, appear to
provide tension reduction for the speaker who is uttering them. They
become more prevalent under the same conditions that a stutterer's
stuttering increases in severity. For example, time pressures, in-
security regarding subject matter, a threatening listener all increase
the amounts of normal disfluency we use. The important factor is
that we use them in a "bubbly" forward moving manner. We tolerate
them and often are comparatively unaware of their presence. In
other words, all of us have periods of primary stuttering.

Most stutterers, I believe, have few if any normal disfluencies in
their speech. Much stuttered speech is characterized by tense repetitions of sounds and syllables and by interjections of non-meaningful
verbalizations, which are not serving as tension reducers, but rather

as avoidances, postponements and starters which build tension, rather
than reduce it! Normal disfluences are often identified by stutterers
as abnormal and when this normal means of tension reduction is inhibited.
tension builds and stuttering occurs.

I suggest that all clinicians should attempt sometime to speak with
complete fluency.   When you attempt it, do not allow yourself an interjection of uh, er, well or mmm. Inhibit all word and phrase repetitions.
Do not allow yourself the privilege of revising your word patterns. Do
not even allow a pause. After a period of time, you will develop tension,
blocking and you will come closer to knowing what true stuttering feels
like than you thought possible.

During the past five years, in addition to other individual and group
therapy approaches, all of the stutterers with whom I have worked,
have been taught to be disfluent in a normal, rather than in an abnormal
manner. This technique, Voluntary Normal Disfluency, will be described
in detail, in the time which remains for my presentation in today's program. It is not offered as a panacea, nor as a solution to all of the
complex problems of those who stutter. It is presented, however, as
a technique that can be used easily without conflict by all clinicians,
regardless of theoretical bias or other therapeutic preferences.

Voluntary Normal Disfluency can best be defined as the purposeful
use of the easy forward moving interruptions that occur in varying
amounts in normal conversational speech. It is an organized, planned

system for developing in the stutterer a feeling of what it is like to be disfluent in a normal, rather than an abnormal way.

Most of us are not aware of our normal disfluencies. If we are to teach stutterers to exhibit them in a normal manner, we must become acutely aware of all aspects of how they are produced by normal speakers. Certain observations are pertinent.

1. Word and phrase repetitions are usually single rather than multiple.

2. They occur most frequently on short words such as prepositions, conjunctions, pronouns, articles and short verbs.

3. They are usually unstressed. In other words, they do not stand out in terms of loudness or pitch.

4. They are produced effortlessly and rapidly.

5. They vary in their frequency of occurrence. There may be many of them in one sentence and none in the next.

A number of observations have led to the development and refinement of normal voluntary disfluency techniques.

1. I have observed repeatedly that stutterers who recover either through therapy or by the route of "spontaneous recovery" exhibit more frequent effortless word and phrase repetitions than those who continue exhibiting stuttering symptoms. (For example, Dr. Joseph Sheehen, who exhibits closer to normal speech than any of the stuttering authorities on stuttering I have heard, has more frequent normal disfluencies than any of the others I have heard.)

2. When stutterers are fluent, they are frequently abnormally
   fluent.

3. During periods of relative fluency many stutterers exhibit
   normal disfluencies that are not present in their stuttered
   speech.

When using Voluntary Normal Disfluency, I suggested that these
general rules be followed:

1. Use primarily in the form of word and phrase repetitions.

2. Use only on non-feared words upon which there is no stuttering. If the stutterer is extremely severe and he has no
   non-feared words, Voluntary Normal Disfluency is delayed.

3. Vary the number of repetitions of words and phrases so that
   no pattern is established. Usually make them single, rather
   than multiple repetitions.

4. Do not use a postponement device when stuttering is anticipated.

5. Use in an effortless manner with no feeling of control or over-
   preciseness.

6. Use at the beginning of phrase or thought groups, so that they
   resemble normal disfluencies. If they occur on the last word
   or group of words, they sound artificial and unnatural.

7. Do not use part-word repetitions or prolongations voluntarily.
   Reserve these for the purpose of approaching and moving
   through actual moments of stuttering.

8. Use first in the speaking or reading situations that is likely to provide the greatest opportunity for free speech for each individual. Utilize the adaptation effect when necessary by using the same material repeatedly until the individual becomes fluent. Then introduce Voluntary Normal Disfluency.

9. If an attempt at Voluntary Normal Disfluency turns into a real moment of stuttering, it should not be treated as a failure, but rather approached as any other moment of stuttering.

10. Do not confuse the situation by using voluntary stuttering. This is usually resisted by stutterers and it has no relation to Voluntary Normal Disfluency.

11. Do not praise moments of spontaneous fluency. Such periods occur in all stutterers, but praising them merely reinforces opposition to the toleration of normal fluency.

12. Clinicians must become aware of their own disfluencies and be able to produce them voluntarily easily during therapy sessions.

13. Include ear-training activities in therapy to build an awareness of how disfluent normal speech really is. Get tapes of the child's parents and siblings, whom he feels have good speech, and point out examples of disfluency. Tapes of radio and television interview shows also provide sources of normal disfluencies.

14. Instruct parents and teachers so that they accept disfluency mistakenly identified as evidence of the stuttering. Some actual speech training of the parent may be in order so that the child's speech environment contains evidences of easy forward moving "bubbled" speech. I make school visits to make certain that the stutterer's teachers and fellow students understand the problem and know how they should respond to it. Normal disfluencies of all children are pointed during these discussions so that the stuttering child's symptoms seem less bizarre.

In conclusion, it should be stated that since Voluntary Normal Disfluency has been included in my therapy plans for stutterers, I have had a higher percentage of complete recoveries, more rapid recoveries, and more stable recoveries without relapse.

Perhaps the best final statement for this paper is the one that concludes my film on voluntary normal disfluency. I suggest that any speech clinician, who feels he or she could be comfortable in using voluntary normal disfluency in conjunction with other therapeutic approaches with stutterers, should try it.

If you have reservations concerning it... or feel that you would use the approach awkwardly, I urge you do not attempt it until you are fully aware of your own disfluencies and have mastered the use of them voluntarily in your own speech.

197